D0038748

NATUROPATHIC HANDBOOK OF HERBAL FORMULAS

Other Titles from Kivakí Press

Sacred Land, Sacred Sex: Rapture of the Deep—
Concerning Deep Ecology and Celebrating Life

Deep Powder Snow: 40 Years of Ecstatic Skiing,
Avalanches, and Earth Wisdom

by Dolores LaChapelle

Look To The Mountain: An Ecology of Indigenous Education
by Gregory Cajete, Ph.D.

Seasons of Change: Growing Through Pregnancy and Birth
by Suzanne Arms

Restoration Forestry: Forestry Practices for a Sustainable Future
Michael Pilarski, Ed.

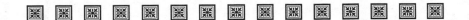

NATUROPATHIC HANDBOOK OF HERBAL FORMULAS

A Practical and Concise Herb User's Guide

Richard Scalzo

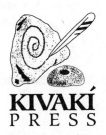

KIVAKÍ
PRESS

Acknowledgments

I would like to acknowledge the teachers who have inspired me in both subjective and objective paths of gaining knowledge, and who have motivated me to think deeply about the relationships that exist between humans and plants. I would also like to acknowledge the many naturopathic physicians with whom my path has crossed, including Drs. Bill Mitchell and Ed Madison. I am also grateful for the technical writing support of Cynthia Baddour and the publishing efforts of Greg Cumberford at Kivakí Press. And finally, I wish to acknowledge the inspiration and wisdom that I have received from the plant kingdom.

Copyright ©1994 Richard Scalzo

All rights reserved. No part of this book may be reproduced in any form or by any electronic or mechanical means, including information storage and retrieval systems, except for brief reviews, without permission in writing from the publisher.

Kivakí Press
585 East 31st Street
Durango, Colorado 81301
(303) 385-1767

Publisher's Cataloging in Publication

Scalzo, Richard.
   Naturopathic handbook of herbal formulas : a practical and concise herb user's guide / Richard Scalzo. — 3rd ed.
   p. cm.
   ISBN 1-882308-42-5

   1. Herbs—Therapeutic use. 2. Naturopathy.   I. Title.

   RM666.H33S35 1994   615.321
                                       QBI93-503

Third Edition
First Printing, 1994

Printed in the United States of America
3 4 5 6 7 — 98 97 96 95 94

TABLE OF CONTENTS

NATUROPATHIC HANDBOOK OF HERBAL FORMULAS

A PRACTICAL & CONCISE HERB USER'S GUIDE

In each century since the beginning of the world wonderful things have been discovered. In the last century more amazing things were found out than in any century before. In this new century hundreds of things still more astounding will be brought to light. At first, people refuse to believe that a strange new thing can be done, then they begin to hope it can be done, then they see it can be done—then it is done and all the world wonders why it was not done centuries ago.

Frances Hodgson Burnett
from *The Secret Garden*

"ONLY A NEW SEED WILL YIELD A NEW CROP"

Every now and then one comes across opportunities to make decisions which change the course of one's life. During this time, we are witnessing a vast change in society's attitudes and approaches to health and healing. I offer this document for those who recognize the need for this change and for those who are eager to explore the possibilities that it brings.

THE ESSENCE OF ALL BEINGS IS EARTH. THE ESSENCE OF THE EARTH IS WATER. THE ESSENCE OF WATER IS PLANTS. THE ESSENCE OF PLANTS IS THE HUMAN BEING.

Upanishads

BALANCE IN NATURE:
A Wholistic Perspective
On the Use of
Medicinal Plants

Modern medicine is just now on the verge of discovering a unified field that is the deepest level of nature. Ancient cultures have been aware of this dynamic field for thousands of years. It is considered to be the unexpressed wellspring of intelligence within nature that nourishes and fortifies the infinite diversity expressed in life.

All the laws of nature are contained within this unified field in their seed form. As these impulses of nature flower from their seed form, the intelligence or "mind" of nature becomes expressed in the growth and evolution of every living structure. The life cycle of every plant is governed by these fundamental forces of nature, which have been identified by ancient systems of medicine as earth, air, fire, and water. These building blocks of nature have been recognized respectively by modern chemistry as carbon, oxygen, nitrogen, and hydrogen.

It is through the influence and interaction of these "building blocks" with the plant, that the unexpressed pure intelligence of nature is actually metabolized by the tissues and cells of the plant. The mechanics of this are nothing short of amazing. When a seed changes from its dormant phase to its growth phase, the organizing power of nature within the seed structures the correct balance of earth, air, fire, and water, and orchestrates every phase of development of the plant. Through the process of natural selection the plant organizes the various elemental substances in the soil as well as the elemental values or building blocks of nature into its structure. This is the organizing power of nature at work.

When the human physiology metabolizes a plant remedy, it actually metabolizes the organizing power of nature which the plant has transmuted into material form. In this simple way, the human physiology responds to and is governed by the physiology of nature, resulting in the harmonizing of the body and mind of human life with the "body" and "mind" of nature. The specific value of intelligence and order that is expressed in the cells of the plant is metabolized and expressed into the cells of the physiology.

THE VALUE OF PLANTS IN HEALTH AND HEALING

The metabolism of nature's intelligence by human physiology takes place on the level of the neuroreceptors, which serve as a link between the body and the environment. The human body has a multitude of neuroreceptors that respond to complimentary biological substances found in nature. Medicinal plants are capable of targeting specific receptors within the body. In this way, the health and balance of the body is restored by the chemistry and organizing power of the plant. Through the plant's influence, we can greatly enhance our ability to "stitch together" the diverse fabrics of our physiology into a more unified whole.

PLANTS & HOLISTIC MEDICINE:
Whole Plant Extracts vs. Standardized Extracts vs. Common Drugs

Every culture has a history of using plants for healing. At the turn of the century, pharmaceutical practices provided techniques for "standardizing" and "purifying" medicines by isolating active constituents from plants. In today's allopathic medicine, most remedies are synthetic preparations devoid of any life-promoting vital energies. Thus we have witnessed the crude side effects which common drugs have on the physiology.

Traditional herbal medicine has revealed a deep wisdom that modern medicine is just beginning to appreciate. In today's herbal pharmaceutical practices it is well known that every plant requires specific extraction methods to yield the strongest and most vital remedy. For example, some plants are best prepared by boiling for several hours, while others are best prepared by infusing into cold water. Some plants require fermentation, while others need acidifying. Some are best extracted in oil, while others are best extracted in pure grain alcohol. Traditional practices and modern research guide us in the proper methods of preparing plant remedies. The art of preparing a plant remedy lies in knowing about and working with the "mind" and the "body" of the plant to bring forth its healing virtues.

Common drugs and standardized herbal remedies do not have the wholistic effect within the body that whole plant extracts do. Standardized herbal preparations favor one active constituent of a plant. Common drugs provide a chemical similar to an active constituent. Both can have strong effects but always at the expense of the whole. In contrast, whole plant extracts, artfully and scientifically prepared, provide the most complete range of the plant's chemistry and synergy and therefore exercise the most wholistic influence on the physiology.

THE VALUE OF FRESHNESS IN MEDICINAL PLANT PREPARATIONS

Herbal preparations are only as vital as the plants used to prepare the remedy. An effective herbal extract should capture the essence of nature's vitality and resemble the plant in taste, smell, and color.

In order to achieve these results, fresh living plants used for extraction are best. When a plant is still fresh and succulent, its cells are naturally swollen and most capable of releasing their therapeutic qualities into the extraction menstruum. This is especially true when using plants that rely on volatile oils for their effectiveness. Volatile oils are aromatic and susceptible to depreciation when exposed to drying, storage, heat, or light. A good fresh–plant extract of peppermint, for example, should have that rich flavor, taste, and smell which one experiences when chewing a fresh peppermint leaf.

In many cases the degree to which plants are dried proportionally depreciates the active, volatile constituents of the plant. Fresh plants are also rich in enzymes which may catalyze the therapeutic constituents of the plant, enabling them to be most wholistic in their action upon the body.

There are, however, some exceptions to this principle of freshness. Plants that have very strong organic fixed principles, resins, gums, and seeds, as well as plants that are cathartic in their action, must be dried before extraction. In the case of cathartic plants, drying and aging the plant renders the activity less irritating. In many cases the properties of herbs are altered by drying the plant. One good example is ginger root. In its fresh state, ginger root is warming and diffusive, rather gentle in its action. In its dry state, ginger root is hot and direct, very strong in its action.

Perhaps the best approach to take in preparing herbal extracts is one that enables the extract to mirror the fresh plant as closely as possible. With correct extraction methods, fresh plant extracts appear to accomplish this goal most successfully.

EXTRACTION TECHNIQUES: Defining the Terms Used

In herbal pharmacy there are many methods of preparing herbal extracts. Below are definitions of the terms used in the common preparations of herbal remedies. *(Please note: These are very condensed descriptions.)*

Tinctures—An alcoholic or hydro-alcoholic preparation providing a dry herb strength ratio of 1:5. Thus, tinctures represent an herb strength of one part herb for every five parts extract.

Liquid Extracts—An alcoholic or hydro-alcoholic

preparation generally providing a dry or fresh herb strength ratio of 1:2. Liquid extracts are fully saturated preparations representing an herb strength of one part herb for every two parts extract.

U.S. Pharmacopoeia Fluid Extracts—An alcoholic or hydro-alcoholic preparation providing a dry herb strength ratio of 1:1. This means U.S. Pharmacopoeia Fluid Extracts represent a dry herb strength of one part herb for every part extract. In order to accomplish this concentration, special extraction methods and equipment are necessary involving heat and vacuum.

Fresh Plant Fluid Extracts—An alcoholic or hydro-alcoholic preparation providing a fresh herb strength ratio of 1:1. Fresh Plant Fluid Extracts provide one part herb by weight for every part menstruum by volume. Thus Fresh Plant Fluid Extracts utilize a weight/volume ratio which takes into account the moisture content within the fresh plant.

Solid Extracts—An evaporated U.S. Pharmacopoeia Fluid Extract concentrated by evaporation or vacuum extraction to a dry herb ratio of 4:1. This represents four parts herb for every part of extract.

Powdered Extracts—A powdered version of a U.S. Pharmacopoeia Fluid Extract or Solid Extract. These extracts are prepared by evaporation methods to remove all liquids. The concentration ratio of powdered extracts may vary ranging from 1:1 to 10:1 or stronger.

Standardized Extracts—A powdered extract prepared by methods described above. However, these extracts represent a significantly higher, "standardized" level of the major active constituent within the herb. Some standardized extracts are "standardized" by identifying an active constituent and guaranteeing a consistent level of the constituent in the preparation. In this case, no alteration of the ratio of constituents within the plant takes place.

A COMMENT ON HERBAL USAGE

When using herbs, it is wise to determine whether the compound is to be used therapeutically or tonically. If an herb is to be used therapeutically, it is best to use it for a short period of time (1–4 weeks) at the appropriate time of day or evening. Some herbs are more effective when taken during the morning hours (i.e., Greater Celandine) while others are more effective when taken during the evening hours (i.e., Milk Thistle Seed).

If an herb or compound is to be used tonically (to alter a deep imbalance), it is best to use for a long period of time (4–6 months or longer). For example, Hawthorn Berry, a wonderful cardiovascular tonic, exerts its influence best when used 6–12 months consecutively.

Invariably, one should apply the simple principle of "rest/activity" when using herbs. A general recommendation would be to use herbs six days on and one day off, six weeks on and one week off, six months on and one month off. Each period of rest from herbal usage allows the effects of the herbs to become integrated into the physiology.

A very simple analogy will illustrate this. When one wants to dye a white cloth blue, one dips the cloth in dye and then sets it in the sun to dry. When dry, it is noticeable that some of the color has been lost, yet some remains. Again the cloth is dipped in the dye and set back in the sun to dry. Some color again is lost, but more remains. The alternation of this process of "rest and activity" enables the color to become steadfast. Likewise, periodic days of "rest" from herbal remedies enable the physiology to integrate the effects of the herbal compounds and make those effects permanent.

This principle of rest and activity is a fundamental law of nature which governs all growth and evolution of life. Incorporating this principle into herbal usage greatly simplifies, yet profoundly strengthens, the process of using herbs in the healing arts.

COMPOUNDING HERBS— CREATING SYNERGY

Herbal compounding is the selection of two or more therapeutic plants combined together to benefit the physiology. The ancient herbal systems of Chinese Medicine and Indian Ayurvedic Medicine provide illustrations of this in their materia medicas.

Medicinal plants are compounded to: increase therapeutic effectiveness; alter individual actions of herbs; and minimize or negate any toxic side effects of unusually strong herbs. In Chinese medicine, herbs are compounded to enhance the individual constituents. There is always a primary herb within the compound that represents the thrust of the formula. The other herbs enhance, assist, or direct the primary herb in its action. In Ayurvedic Medicine, herbs are often compounded with metals and minerals to bring out the positive effects and neutralize the toxic effects of stronger herbs.

Herbal compounding invariably creates a synergy which enables the formula to function most effectively. This art and science has been practiced for over 5,000 years and today forms the core of clinical herbalism.

This Dispensatory Guide is intended to assist in the professional use of botanical formulas. It is not intended to replace physician's health care. It is written for educational purposes only. If a medical condition is present, it would be wise to seek the counsel of a professionally trained and licensed naturopathic physician.

COMPOUNDED ARTEMESIA/QUASSIA
An Anti-Parasitic Formula

Contents: Fresh Wormword Herb (Artemesia annua), Quassia Bark (Picaraena excelsa), Fresh Black Walnut Hulls (Juglans nigra), Neem Leaves (Azardica indica), Bilva Herb (Aegle marmelos), Embelia ribes, Eclipta alba, Phallanthus amarus, Gentian Root (Gentiana lutea), Fresh Ginger Root (Zingiber officinalis).

Therapeutic Actions: This compound contains bitter principles which activate secretions of the digestive and alimentary canals. The vermifuge and vermicide activity is strong, acting upon a wide range of worms, amoebas, and parasites.

Indications: This compound is indicated whenever there may be a suspicion of pinworms, ringworms, roundworms, tapeworms, microbial growth and parasitic activity. Also this compound can be used to address fungal and yeast growth, both internally as well as locally.

Uses/Dosage: Take 30–40 drops of this compound 3–5 times daily in a small amount of warm water. While using this compound it would be wise to avoid the foods which parasites and worms thrive upon: sugar, refined carbohydrates, processed foods, etc. Drink plenty of warm water throughout the day to accelerate the effects of these herbs. Use this compound no longer than 3 weeks at a time.

Contra-indications and Cautions:	Do not use this compound during pregnancy or whenever there may be chronic illness present. Modify dosage accordingly for children.

COMPOUNDED ASTRAGALUS
A Deep Immune-Enhancing Formula

Contents:	Chinese Astragalus Root (Astragalus membranicus), Chinese Ligustrum Berry (Ligustrum lucidum), Chinese Schizandra Berry (Schizandra chinensis).
Therapeutic Actions:	This compound targets the body's deepest line of defense. The herbs bring support to all deep immune functions and activate cellular immunity. This compound may be used therapeutically for chronic conditions as well as tonically for deep immune support.
Indications:	Use these herbs when there is chronic immune deficiency or breakdown of the deep immune functions. Use as an adjunct in the treatment of cancer, AIDS, arthritis, lupus, blood disorders, anemia, amenorrhea, Epstein-Barr Virus (EBV). This compound may also be used when there are recurring cold/flu infections which prevail chronically throughout the winter.
Uses/Dosage:	Take 30–40 drops of the compound 3–5 times daily in a small amount of warm water. Best results are achieved when used for 4–6 months or longer. If chronic cold/flu syndrome is present, do not use this compound during acute cold symptoms.

Complementary Compounds:	This compound is compatible with other deep plant adaptogens such as Siberian Ginseng and Compounded Rejuvenative Elixir, as well as Compounded Elixir of Siberian Ginseng and Reishi Mushroom.

COMPOUNDED BLOODROOT/CELANDINE
An Anti Retro-Viral Compound

Contents:	Fresh Bloodroot (Sanguinaria canadensis), Fresh Celandine Flowering Tops (Chelidonium major), Prickly Ash Bark (Xanthoxylum clava-herculis).
Therapeutic Actions:	This compound contains potent alkaloids which target the category of viruses known as retro-viruses. These alkaloids exhibit an inhibitory effort upon the reverse transcriptase enzyme which is the enzyme used by retro-viruses to transcribe the viral genetics into the genetics of the human cell. This compound may be an effective tool in the management of retro-viral infections.
Indications:	This compound is used to manage the progression of retro-viruses at the genetic level of the cell. Retro-viruses include HIV, Epstein-Barr (EBV), Mononucleosis, and Herpes.
Uses/Dosage:	Take 10–15 drops of this compound 3–4 times daily in a small amount of warm water. Use for 2 weeks, then discontinue use for 2 weeks. If opportunistic infection is present use the complementary herbs cited below.
Complementary Compounds:	Add to the above compound Fresh Thuja extract (for 2 weeks only), Compounded Astragalus, Fresh St. John's Wort Extract, Licorice Root Solid Extract, Compounded Lomatium and Reishi Mushroom Extract.
Contra-indications and Cautions:	Do not use this compound during pregnancy. Do not take this compound for longer than 2 weeks

consecutively as the alkaloids may cause liver distress.

COMPOUNDED BUGLEWEED/MOTHERWORT
An Over-Active Thyroid Compound

Contents: Fresh Bugleweed Herb (Lycopus virginica), Fresh Motherwort Flowering Tops (Leonurus cardiaca), Fresh Lemon Balm Herb (Melissa officinalis).

Therapeutic Actions: This compound targets the thyroid stimulating hormone and may normalize a hyperactive thyroid condition.

Indications: This compound is used for an over-active thyroid associated with symptoms of excessive metabolism, cardiac distress/cardiac neuroses, palpitations, fatigue, anxiety, weight loss.

Uses/Dosage: Take 30–40 drops of this compound 3–4 times daily in a small amount of warm water. This compound may be taken for 3–4 months then discontinued for one month.

Contra-indications and Cautions: Hyperactive thyroid condition may indicate a more serious health imbalance. It is important to consult your health care provider if there is any question regarding the nature of this imbalance.

COMPOUNDED DANDELION/FENNEL
A Digestive Cordial Compound

Contents: Fresh Dandelion Root & Leaf (Taraxacum officinalis), Fennel Seed (Foeniculum vulgare), Gentian Root (Gentiana leutea), Fresh Peppermint Leaf (Mentha piperita), Licorice Root (Glycyrrhiza glabra), Fresh Ginger Root (Zingiber officinalis).

Therapeutic Actions: This compound contains bitter principles that activate digestive secretions and enriches enzymatic activity upon food metabolism. Also, carminative herbs provide a soothing influence that dispels wind and gases accumulated in the stomach and intestines. This compound may also be used as a tonic for restoring digestive functions.

Indications: This compound is used for abnormal digestive secretions, hypochloridia, gall bladder and liver congestion and stagnation, bloating and abdominal distention, excessive gas in the intestinal tract, abnormal appetite, excess heat in the liver and blood. The pleasant taste of this compound makes it an enjoyable cordial to take after meals to lighten the influences of heavy foods and post digestive heaviness.

Uses/Dosage: Take 30–40 drops of this compound 3 times daily in a small amount of warm water after meals. These herbs may be taken for 4–6 months consecutively.

COMPOUNDED DEVIL'S CLAW/CHAPARRAL
An Anti-Arthritic Formula

Contents: Devil's Claw Root (Harpagophytum procumbens), Chaparral Leaf (Larrea tridentata), Fresh Compounded Echinacea (Echinacea spp.), Fresh Burdock Root & Seed (Arctium lappa), Fresh Black Cohosh Root (Cimicifuga racemosa), Licorice Root (Glycyrrhiza glabra), Prickly Ash Bark (Xanthoxylum clava-herculis).

Therapeutic Actions: This compound contains anti-inflammatory, antioxidant, and immune-enhancing compounds which act to relieve the inflammatory activities associated with arthritic rheumatism.

Indications: As this is a compound that alleviates inflammation of tissues and muscles, specific indications for this compound include muscular rheumatism, and degenerative arthritis associated with deficient immune functions. This compound may also be used for tissue injury manifesting acute inflammations.

Complementary Compounds:

As a broad and comprehensive approach to arthritis, it is suggested that this compound be used with Compounded Red Clover and Compounded Juniper Berry for general tissue and blood alteration. For additional support, herbal salicylates found in Willow Bark and Meadowsweet are very useful as well as Compounded Turmeric/Catechu which contains natural flavonoids to promote tissue integrity and greater anti-oxidant activity.

Uses/Dosage:

Take 30–40 drops 3–4 times daily in a small amount of warm water between meals. This compound and its complementary compounds should be taken for 6 months or longer to effect a good result.

COMPOUNDED DONG QUAI
A Female Hormonal Balancing Formula

Contents:

Chinese Dong Quai Root (Angelica sinensis), Helonias Root (Chamoelirium leuteum), Fresh Black Cohosh Root (Cimicifuga racemosa), Fresh Squaw Vine (Mitchella repens), Fresh Saw Palmetto Berry (Serenoa repens), Licorice Root (Glycyrrhiza glabra), Fresh Ginger Root (Zingiber officinalis).

Therapeutic Actions:

This compound targets the ovaries and uterus and lends both a nourishing and tonifying influence to these organs. The herbs exert a balancing effect upon the hormonal functions pertaining to the monthly cycle.

Indications:

As a hormonal balancing compound, dysfunctions relating to hormonal imbalances are addressed with this compound. It is effective in correcting the problems of amenorrhea (absence of or delayed menses), dysmenorrhea (painful menstruation), menorrhagia (excessive menstrual bleeding), and metrorrhagia (excessive uterine bleeding). This compound may also be used to address painful ovulation or ovarian pain, as well as an adjunct therapy in the treatment of endometriosis. Also useful for pelvic atony and prolapsed pelvic organs.

Complementary Compounds: This compound is synergistic with Compounded Elixir of Vitex and can be used by alternately taking Compounded Dong Quai during the follicular phase (day 1–14) of the cycle and Compounded Elixir of Vitex during the luteal phase (day 14–28) of the cycle.

Uses/Dosage: Take 30-40 drops 3 times daily in a small amount of warm water between meals. Take at least 4-6 months for corrective therapy or as a tonic for the entire reproductive system.

Specific Differentiations: For dysmenorrhea use with Compounded Feverfew/ Jamaican Dogwood. For menorrhagia use with extracts of Yarrow, Shepherd's Purse, and Goldenseal.

COMPOUNDED DEVIL'S CLUB
A Blood Sugar Balancing Formula

Contents: Fresh Devil's Club Root Bark (Oplopanax horridum), Jambul Seed (Syzgium jambolana), Fresh Dandelion Root & Leaf (Taraxacum officinalis), Fresh Uva Ursi Leaf (Arctostaphylos uva ursi), Fresh Turmeric Root (Curcuma longa).

Therapeutic Actions: This compound acts upon the re-synthesis of glycogen, facilitates in the repair of the isles of langerhan of the pancreas, and promotes better production and utilization of insulin. Since this is a balancing compound, its action is to normalize and restore integrity of the organs and glands associated with carbohydrate and sugar metabolism.

Indications: These herbs are indicated in both hyper- and hypoglycemia. Use as an adjunct to the daily diet for promoting a greater balance of glucose metabolism within the body.

Complementary Compounds: In both hyper- and hypoglycemia it is useful to use this compound along with Compounded Elixir of Bitters, which promotes a greater balance to the digestive functions.

Uses/Dosage: Take 30-40 drops of extract and add to a small amount of warm water. Take shortly before meals, 3 times daily. Continue to use this compound for 3–4 months.

Contra-indications and Cautions: This compound should not be taken during pregnancy and should not necessarily be considered a substitute for insulin therapy.

COMPOUNDED ECHINACEA
An Anti-Viral and Secretory Immune Formula

Contents: Fresh Echinacea angustifolia Root, Fresh Echinacea purpurea Root, Fresh Echinacea purpurea Flowering Heads, Ripe Echinacea purpurea Seed.

Therapeutic Actions: This compound targets the secretory immune system (lymph system, skin, and mucous membranes) and activates cellular immunity when the cellular integrity is threatened by viral attack. This compound also contains anti–inflammatory activity, interferon–like activity, and promotes the production of fibroblasts for wound healing.

Indications: Echinacea is used most effectively at the onset of secretory viral infections and used in large doses. Specific indications include: sinus, nasal, ear, and throat infections; respiratory tract infections; lymphatic infections; lymphatic swelling; kidney, bladder, and urinary tract infections; ovarian and prostate infections. Other indications for its use include inflammatory arthritis, toxemia of the blood, wounds, and cancers of the secretory tissues. Specifically indicated for the common cold and flu-type viral infections.

Complementary Compounds: Echinacea may be used compatibly in the treatment of secretory immune conditions with diaphoretic herbs such as yarrow, elder flowers, peppermint, ginger, sage, and boneset. Other compatible herbs include secretory immune modulators such as prickly ash bark and spilanthes.

Uses/Dosage: At the onset of viral infection, add 2–3 teaspoons of Echinacea extract to a small amount of warm water and take as an initial dose. Then follow with subsequent doses of 1–2 teaspoons of Echinacea extract every 2 hours and take for up to 5 days. Children's dose should be modified to 5 drops of extract for every year of age until the adult dose is reached.

COMPOUNDED ECHINACEA/GOLDENSEAL
An Anti-Viral/Anti-Bacterial/Antibiotic Compound

Contents: Fresh Echinacea spp., Fresh Goldenseal Root (Hydrastis canadensis), Fresh Oregon Grape Root (Berberis aquafolium), Fresh Barberry Root Bark (Berberis vulgaris), Fresh St. John's Wort Flowering Buds (Hypericum perforatum), Propolis (Bee-harvested Tree Resin).

Therapeutic Actions: This compound contains active alkaloids which act as strong natural antibiotics effective in the treatment of a broad spectrum of bacterial conditions. Microbials which this compound addresses directly include Staph spp., Strep. spp., Chlamydia spp., E. Coli, Salmonella, Giardia, Trichomonas, and Candida yeast. The anti-viral properties of this compound address a broad spectrum of viral conditions including secretory viruses and retro-viruses.

Indications: This compound is indicated for the above cited microbials and viruses. At the onset of viral infection it is recommended in frequent and large doses. It is also indicated in the treatment of the common cold and flu viruses, and for infections of the lymphatic system. It may also be used externally as a wash for wounds, cuts, and abrasions as well as for insect bites and bee stings.

Complementary Compounds: For chronic immune imbalances use with deeper-acting immune enhancers such as Compounded Astragalus, Siberian Ginseng, and Siberian Ginseng Tonic.

Contra-indications and Cautions: This product should not be used during pregnancy. Prolonged and large doses of Goldenseal may disturb the balance of micro-flora in the gut and the intestines.

Dosage: At the onset of viral and bacterial infections, take an initial dose of 2–3 teaspoons of extract in a small amount of warm water. Follow with subsequent doses of 1–2 teaspoons in warm water every 2 hours for a maximum of 5 days.

COMPOUNDED ECHINACEA/RED ROOT
A Blood & Lymphatic Alterative Compound

Contents: Fresh Echinacea spp., Fresh Red Root (Ceanothus americanus), Fresh Baptisia Root (Baptisia tinctoria), Fresh Thuja Leaf (Thuja occidentalis), Fresh Stillingia Root (Stillingia sylvatica), Fresh Blue Flag Root (Iris versicolor), Prickly Ash Bark (Xanthoxylum clava-herculus).

Therapeutic Actions: The herbs within this compound act as blood and lymphatic alteratives and bring about distinct and definite changes in metabolism-repairing catabolic tissue and waste. This compound also augments the body's natural defense mechanisms by activating natural immune responses.

Indications: These herbs are indicated for conditions associated with a buildup of catabolic wastes in the tissues. Specifically indicated for cancers, tumor growths, incipient cancers, blood dyscrasias, lymphatic engorgement, cysts, fluid cysts, ovarian cysts, endometriosis, cervical dysplasia, and skin ulcerations. Also indicated for those conditions which are associated with a breakdown of the auto-immune system.

Complementary Compounds: Compounded Echinacea/Goldenseal.

Dosage: Take 20–40 drops of extract in a small amount of warm water 3–5 times daily between meals. Continue using for 2–3 months if necessary.

Contra-indications and Cautions: Do not use this compound during pregnancy. If pathology is present, this compound should not replace medical or alternative medical care.

COMPOUNDED EYEBRIGHT/BAYBERRY
Hay Fever, Allergy & Sinus Compound

Contents: Fresh Eyebright Herb (Euphrasia officinalis), Fresh Bayberry Root (Myrica cerifera), Fresh Goldenseal Root (Hydrastis canadensis), Fresh Calamus Root (Acorus calamus), Fresh Stinging Nettle Leaf (Urtica dioica).

Therapeutic Actions: This compound acts to constringe, condense, and contract the swollen mucous membranes associated with hayfevers and allergies. The astringent and anti-inflammatory actions bring tone and firmness to soggy membranes. Also, anti-bacterial activity enables this formula to check infections associated with the sinus and nasal cavity.

Indications: This compound should be used for the symptomatic relief of hayfever, allergies, and excessive mucous congestion of the sinus, nasal, ear, and throat. Also specifically indicated for sinus infections associated with excessive catarrhal exudations.

Uses/Dosage: Take 30–40 drops of this compound added to a small amount of warm water and take 3–5 times daily until symptoms are relieved.

Complementary Compounds: If sinus infection is present, use compatibly with Compounded Echinacea/Goldenseal.

Contra-indications and Cautions: Do not use this compound if excessive dryness of the mucous tissue is already present. Do not use this compound during pregnancy. This compound is designed for short term use only. Use only until symptoms disappear.

COMPOUNDED FENNEL/WILD YAM
A Gallstone/Fatty Digestion Compound

Contents: Fennel Seed (Foeniculum vulgare), Fresh Wild Yam Root (Dioscorea villosa), Fresh Fringe Tree Root Bark (Chionanthus virginica), Fresh Dandelion Root & Leaf (Taraxacum officinalis), Fresh Celandine Root & Tops (Chelidonium major), Fresh California Poppy (Escholzia californica), Peppermint Oil.

Therapeutic Actions: This compound contains principles which have choleretic and spasmolytic properties that promote the release and the flow of congested bile through the gall system, and that relax the muscles and membranes to alleviate spastic cramps associated with gall bladder colic.

Indications: This compound is indicated for the relief of gall bladder congestion or obstructed gall ducts associated with gall bladder colic, incipient gall stones, and bile stagnation. Individuals who have difficulty digesting fatty and unctuous foods are benefited greatly with this compound.

Complementary Compounds:

The use of Compounded Elixir of Bitters will greatly enhance the actions of this compound.

Uses/Dosage:

Take 30–40 drops of this compound 3–4 times daily in a small amount of warm water either before or after meals.

Contra-indications and Cautions:

Do not use this compound during pregnancy. This compound must be used with great care if gall stones are present. Please consult your health care provider if a medical condition is present.

COMPOUNDED FEVERFEW/ JAMAICAN DOGWOOD
A Headache, Migraine, & Anti-Pain Formula

Contents:

Fresh Feverfew Flowering Herb (Chrysanthemum parthenium), Jamaican Dogwood Bark (Piscidia erythina), Fresh Black Haw Root & Tree Bark (Viburnum prunifolium), Fresh St. John's Wort Flower Buds (Hypericum perforatum), Fresh Butterbur Root (Petasites frigida), Meadowsweet Herb (Filipendula ulmaria), Fresh Willow Bark (Salix spp.), Fresh Ginger Root (Zingiber officinalis).

Therapeutic Actions:

The herbs in this compound act as an anodyne (pain relieving), and an anti-spasmodic. Active principles in these herbs address pain and spasms in all parts of the body.

Indications:

This compound may be used for the relief of pain due to headaches (both tension and migraine headaches), dysmenorrhea (painful menstruation), muscle spasms, muscle/skeletal injuries resulting in pain, intestinal spasms, and painful conditions in the body resulting from chronic arthritis and rheumatism.

Complementary Compounds: For tension headaches, use with Compounded Elixir of Passionflower. For dysmenorrhea, use with Compounded Elixir of Vitex. For muscle/skeletal injuries, use with Compounded Skullcap/St. John's Wort.

Uses/Dosage: For the relief of migraine and tension headaches, it is best to start treatment at the conceptual stage of the headache. Administer 1 teaspoon in a small amount of warm water as an initial dose and follow with subsequent doses of 40–60 drops every 30–60 minutes until pain is relieved. It is wise to rest during this administration time to facilitate the actions of the herbs. For dysmenorrhea and other acute pain, take 40–60 drops of extract in a small amount of warm water every 1–2 hours until pain subsides.

COMPOUNDED FRAXINUS/CEANOTHUS
A Uterine Fibroid and Cyst Corrective Compound

Contents: Fresh Mt. Ash Bark (Fraxinus americanus), Fresh Red Root (Ceanothus americanus), Fresh Life Root (Senecio aurus), Fresh Dandelion Root (Taraxacum officinalis), Fresh Helonias Root (Chamaelirium luteum), Fresh Goldenseal Root (Hydrastis canadensis), Fresh Ginger Root (Zingiber officinalis).

Therapeutic Actions: The herbs in this compound act to remove catabolic wastes from the pelvic cavity, and from uterine and ovarian tissues. These herbs accelerate metabolism and lymph drainage and promote the sloughing-off of wasted tissues.

Indications: This compound is indicated for the treatment of uterine fibroids, ovarian cysts and endometriosis, as well as uterine atony, prolapsed pelvic organ, and stagnation of the pelvic viscera.

Complementary Compounds:	For the treatment of uterine fibroids, ovarian cysts, and endometriosis, this compound should be used with Compounded Scudder's Alterative, Compounded Echinacea/Red Root, and Compounded Gelsemium/Phytolacca.★ If tissue tension is present in the uterine region, use with Black Cohosh Root as well.
Uses/Dosage:	Use 40–60 drops of this extract in a small amount of warm water and take 3–4 times daily for up to 3–4 months.
Contra-indications and Cautions:	Do not use this compound during pregnancy. ★ *Use only under direct physician's care as the asterisk compound cited above may be toxic if not used properly.*

COMPOUNDED GELSEMIUM/PHYTOLACCA
An Ovarian Cyst Compound

Contents:	Fresh Gelsemium Root (Gelsemium sempervirens), Fresh Poke Root (Phytolacca americana) Fresh Aconite (Aconitum napellus), Bryonia Root (Bryonia dioica).
Therapeutic Actions:	The herbs in this compound are considered to be very strong and potentially toxic if misused. They act to dislodge and slough off catabolic waste tissue and promote the drainage of lymphatic fluids from areas affected by the buildup of wastes.
Indications:	This compound is used specifically for the treatment of ovarian cysts and endometriosis. Other uses include severe, irritating, explosive cough, and pain associated with tension and tenderness.
Uses/Dosage:	Take 5–8 drops of the compound in a small amount of warm water 2–3 times daily for up to 2 weeks. *Use only under the care of a licensed naturopathic physician.*

Contra-indications and Cautions: Do not use this compound during pregnancy. Do not use with children. This compound may be toxic if used incorrectly.

 COMPOUNDED GINSENG/SCHIZANDRA
An Adrenal/Adaptogenic Compound

Contents: Siberian Ginseng Root (Eleutherococcus senticossus), Chinese Schizandra Berry (Schizandra chinensis), Damiana Leaf (Turnera diffusa), Cola Nut (Cola nitida), Fresh Wild Oats (Avena sativa), Licorice Root (Glycyrrhiza glabra), Fresh Skullcap Herb (Scutellaria lateriflora), Prickly Ash Bark (Xanthoxylum clava-herculis).

Therapeutic Actions: The herbs in this compound act to restore integrity to the adrenal glands and promote a greater sense of energy and stamina. The adaptogenic properties of these herbs help to build up the body's response to stress. These herbs are also nutritive and tonic to the adrenal glands as well as to nerve cells and tissues.

Indications: This compound is indicated as an adjunct therapy in the treatment of Addison's Disease (an adrenal deficient disorder). Also specifically indicated for those exhibiting low adrenal function which manifests into low vitality, anemia, low blood pressure, anxiety, physical strain and pressure, and low and depleted energy. As an adaptogen, this compound is very useful for those who are constantly exposed to stressful environments or situations, overwork, excess strain to mind and body, and those involved in weight management and bodybuilding programs.

Complementary Compounds: Use this compound with Siberian Ginseng Tonic, Compounded Smilax/Damiana, or Compounded Elixir of Eleutherox whenever the indications call for any of these compounds.

Uses/Dosage:	Take 30–40 drops of the extract 3–4 times daily in a small amount of warm water between meals. Use for 3–4 months consecutively for best results.
Contra-indications and Cautions:	Do not use this compound during pregnancy. Do not use this compound if there are conditions present associated with hyper-adrenalism.

COMPOUNDED WILD GINSENG
An Energy, Anti-Stress, & Adaptogenic Compound

Contents:	Wild Siberian Ginseng Root (Eleutherococcus senticosus), Fresh Wild American Ginseng Root (Panax Quinquifolium).
Therapeutic Actions:	This compound is a classic adaptogenic formula which helps the body adapt to stressful environments and situations more efficiently. The eleutherosides and ginsinosides in this compound have a positive influence upon all major organs and glands, improving the vitality and stamina of the entire psychophysiological system.
Indications:	This compound may be used as a tonic to improve stamina, endurance, energy, and vitality. Specifically indicated where the adrenals are exhausted and the endocrine functions are at a low ebb. Use as a restorative and energizing tonic when stress levels are high.
Complementary Compounds:	To improve energy and vitality, this compound may be used with Compounded Rejuvenative Elixir and Siberian Ginseng Tonic. When there is mental stress it may be used with Compounded Gotu Kola and Ginkgo extracts.
Uses/Dosage:	Take 10–20 drops of this compound in a small amount of warm water 3 times daily. Best results are achieved if taken for 3–4 months consecutively.

Contra-indications and Cautions:	Do not take this compound during pregnancy. If cardiac conditions are present, this compound should only be used under care by a naturopathic physician.

COMPOUNDED GLYCONDA CORDIAL
An Herbal Antacid and Heartburn Remedy

Contents:	Turkey Rhubarb Root (Rheum palmatum), Fresh Goldenseal Root (Hydrastis canadensis), Cinnamon Bark (Cinnamomum zeylandicum), Peppermint Essential Oil, Potassium Bicarbonate, Vegetable Glycerine.
Therapeutic Actions:	This compound targets the upper gastric system and is traditionally used as an herbal alternative to antacids. It has alterative effects on the upper GI tract and is useful for both diarrhea and constipation. This pleasant-tasting formula may be combined with bad tasting remedies for administration to children.
Indications:	Use this compound as an alternative to Tums or Rolaids whenever acid indigestion is present. Especially effective for gastritis, heartburn, indigestion, belching, and a feeling of heaviness in the esophagus and stomach.
Uses/Dosage:	Take 40–60 drops in a small amount of warm water or soda water after meals or whenever acid indigestion is present.

COMPOUNDED GOTU KOLA
A Memory and Mental Adaptogen Compound

Contents:	Fresh Gotu Kola Leaf and Root (Centella asiatica), Russian Siberian Ginseng (Eleutherococcus senticosus), Fresh Ginkgo Leaf (Ginkgo biloba), Fresh Wild Oats (Avena sativa), Chinese Fo-Ti (He Shou Wu–Polygonum multiflorum), Fresh Peppermint Leaf (Mentha piperita), Rosemary Leaf (Rosmarinus officinalis).

Therapeutic Actions:	The herbs in this compound have anti-oxidant properties which slow down mental aging. Specific actions include improvement to cerebral circulation, peripheral circulation, blood and oxygen supply to the brain, as well as action to reduce the impact which stress has upon the brain and nervous system. Folklore suggests that many of the herbs in this compound directly retard aging of brain and nerve cells.
Indications:	This compound is indicated for short term memory loss, Alzheimer's disease, mental stress and fatigue, impaired peripheral circulation, mental chatter, lack of mental clarity, nervous exhaustion, low adaptive response, and a negative response to stress in general. Use as a general restorative tonic to improve the vitality of the functions of the brain and nerve cells.
Complementary Compounds:	This compound may be used compatibly with Siberian Ginseng Tonic, Compounded Rejuvenative Elixir, and Compounded Elixir of Passionflower.
Uses/Dosage:	Take 30–40 drops of this compound 3–4 times daily in a small amount of warm water between meals. Best results are achieved if used for 3–4 months consecutively.
Contra-indications and Cautions:	This compound should not be used during pregnancy.

COMPOUNDED HAWTHORN
A Cardiovascular & Connective Tissue Compound

Contents:	Hawthorn Berry Solid Extract, Fresh Hawthorn Leaf & Flower (Crataegus oxycantha).
Therapeutic Actions:	This compound contains two groups of active flavonoids which exert their actions upon the heart/cardiovascular system and a second group upon the connective tissue. This compound is regarded as a

cardiovascular tonic, bringing micro-nutrition and microchemistry to the heart and surrounding arteries and capillaries. It is a true restorative to the cardiovascular system. The connective tissue flavonoids act to reinforce the collagen tissue with cross fibers which strengthen this tissue and promotes more vitality to this component of the immune system.

Indications:

This compound is used for rhythmical disturbances of the heart (palpitations, arrhythmias, tachycardia, and cardiac neurosis). Also specifically indicated for myocardial degeneration and acute myocardial insufficiency, cardiac weakness after infections, mitral valve prolapse, elevated cholesterol, hypertension, hypotension, and fatty degeneration of the heart. Other uses include connective tissue support in the treatment of spinal subluxations, inability to hold spinal adjustments, hernias, hemorrhoids, varicosities, prolapsed organs, collagen deficient disorders, and other disorders of the connective tissue.

Complementary Compounds:

This compound may be used effectively with Hawthorn Berry Solid Extract.

Uses/Dosage:

Add 40–60 drops of extract to a small amount of warm water and take 3–5 times daily between meals. Best results are achieved if taken over a 6–12 month period consecutively.

Contra-indications and Cautions:

Do not discontinue the use of this compound abruptly.

COMPOUNDED HOXSEY/RED CLOVER
A Blood & Liver Alterative Compound

Contents:

Fresh Red Clover Blossoms (Trifolium pratense), Buckthorn Bark (Rhamnus cathartica), Fresh Barberry Root Bark (Berberis vulgaris), Fresh Burdock Root (Arctium lappa), Fresh Stillingia Root

(Stillingia sylvatica), Cascara Sagrada Bark (Rhamnus purshiana), Licorice Root (Glycyrrhiza glabra), Prickly Ash Bark (Xanthoxylum clava-herculis). **Note:** *The species of Cascara mentioned in the original Hoxsey formula was thought to be Cascara amarga* (Sweetia panamensis*), not Cascara Sagrada. Cascara Sagrada is offered as an analogue.*

Therapeutic Actions: The herbs in this compound are considered to be classic alteratives which alter catabolic tissues in the body and bring about a tissue change where old, diseased tissue is replaced with healthy, new, more vital tissue. Traditionally these herbs were known as blood purifiers. They act to enhance metabolic functions and promote greater drainage and elimination through the eliminative organs.

Indications: This compound is indicated for the breakdown and removal of metabolic wastes from the body. Specifically indicated for lymphatic engorgement, tumors, incipient cancers, glandular obstructions, and other chronic disorders. This compound provides antiseptic, anti-tumor, and anti-oxidant activity. It normalizes blood imbalances and activates the clearing and defense mechanisms of the liver.

Complementary Compounds: This compound should be used most effectively with Compounded Juniper Berry and plenty of warm water throughout the day.

Uses/Dosage: Add 30–40 drops of extract to a small amount of warm water and take 3–5 times daily. Best results are achieved if used for 3–4 months consecutively.

Contra-indications and Cautions: Do not use this compound during pregnancy.

COMPOUNDED JUNIPER BERRY
A Urinary Diuretic Formula

Contents: Fresh Juniper Berry (Juniperis communis), Fresh

Spring Horsetail (Equisetum arevense), Fresh Corn Silk (Zea mays), Fresh Goldenrod Flowering Tops (Solidago odora), Fresh Cleavers Herb (Galium aparine), Fresh Marshmallow Root (Althaea officinalis).

Therapeutic Actions: This compound contains diuretic, antiseptic, and emollient principles which act to gently stimulate renal excretions, disinfect the urinary tract, and soothe irritated urinary membranes. This compound also functions as a restorative tonic to the entire urinary system.

Indications: This compound is indicated in the treatment of dropsy from renal suppression, cystic catarrh, renal congestion, enuresis, renal obstructions (gravel, bladder stones, calculi), scalding micturition, irritable bladder, cystitis, nephritis, and inability to urinate freely. This compound stimulates the removal of catabolic wastes from the tissues and encourages elimination via the kidneys.

Complementary Compounds: In alterative therapy "blood cleansing," use with Compounded Red Clover and plenty of warm water.

Uses/Dosage: Add 30–40 drops of extract to a small amount of warm water and take 3–5 times daily between meals. Drink plenty of warm water between doses.

Contra-indications and Cautions: Do not use this compound during pregnancy.

COMPOUNDED LINDEN/CRATAEGUS
A Hypertension Compound

Contents: Fresh Linden Flowers (Tilia spp.), Compounded Fresh Hawthorn (Crataegus oxycantha), Fresh Mistletoe (Viscum flavescens), Fresh Valerian Root (Valeriana officinalis).

Therapeutic Actions: The herbs in this compound exert a hypotensive influence and in time will exhibit an anti-arteriosclerotic influence through the absorption of arterial plaque from the walls of the arteries leading to and from the heart.

Indications: Use this compound in the treatment of essential hypertension, high blood pressure, vascular fragility, and cardiac distress. May also be useful with associated conditions such as arteriosclerosis and high cholesterol.

Complementary Compounds: To the above compound add Compounded Hawthorn and Dandelion Root & Leaf to accentuate the effect of the compound. If under the care of a fully licensed naturopathic physician, Rauwolfia Root may also be used (with great caution).

Uses/Dosage: Add 30–40 drops of extract to a small amount of warm water and take 3–4 times daily between meals. Continue to use for 3–4 months for best results.

Contra-indications and Cautions: Do not use this compound during pregnancy.

COMPOUNDED LOBELIA/CALAMUS
A Stop-Smoking Compound

Contents: Fresh Lobelia Herb & Seed (Lobelia inflata), Fresh Calamus Root (Acorus calamus), Fresh Wild Oat Seed (Avena sativa), Fresh St. John's Wort Flower Buds (Hypericum perforatum), Fresh Licorice Root (Glycyrrhiza glabra), Fresh Passionflower Herb (Passiflora incarnata).

Therapeutic Actions: The active principle of this compound, lobeline, is an alkaloid extracted from the Lobelia plant. This alkaloid greatly reduces the desire to ingest nicotine, as the body recognizes the two chemicals in a similar way. Also the adjunct herbs in this compound promote the detoxification of nicotine residues and promote the restoration of the nerve cells and nerve tissues which may have been damaged due to prolonged cigarette smoking.

Indications: This compound is indicated for the individuals who wish to break their smoking habit and at the same time clear out residues left from smoking while restoring important neurological and adrenal functions. To assist in the repair of the nervous system, use Compounded Elixir of Passionflower and Compounded Elixir of Calcium for 3–4 months.

Uses/Dosage: Add 20–30 drops of extract to a small amount of warm water and take 3–4 times daily or more frequently between meals. Continue for 3–4 months for best results.

Contra-indications and Cautions: Do not use this compound during pregnancy. If vomiting occurs due to the emetic property of Lobelia, reduce the dose to $1/2$ the suggested dose.

COMPOUNDED LOMATIUM
An Anti-Viral Compound

Contents: Fresh Lomatium Root (Lomatium dissectum), Fresh Echinacea (Echinacea spp.), Fresh Spilanthes Flowering Herb and Root (Spilanthes acmella), Fresh St. John's Wort Flowering Buds (Hypericum perforatum), Chinese Skullcap Root (Scutellaria baicalensis), Chinese Schizandra Berry (Schizandra chinensis), Licorice Root (Glycyrrhiza glabra), Essential Oil of Cinnamon.

Therapeutic Actions: This compound contains strong anti-viral activity and immune-enhancing properties. Many of the herbs in this compound target cellular immunity and liver functions and act to protect the healthy cells from viral infection, as well as promote a better flow of the vital force through the liver system.

Indications: Specifically indicated in the treatment of chronic viral infection including Epstein-Barr Virus (EBV), hepatitis, shingles, mononucleosis, and other liver viruses. This compound is also indicated as an adjunct in the treatment of Candida Yeast overgrowth and fungal infections as well as herpes infections.

Complementary Compounds: Compounded Echinacea/Goldenseal may be used with the above compound during acute infections. For deeper immune support when there is chronic infection, use with Compounded Astragalus. If there is fungal and yeast overgrowth, use with Compounded Elixir of Bitters and Compounded Spilanthes.

Uses/Dosage: Add 30–40 drops of extract to a small amount of warm water and take 3–4 times daily between meals. For best results, take 3–4 months consecutively.

Contra-indications and Cautions: Do not use this compound during pregnancy. If a skin rash appears from the use of this compound, discontinue its use. Although this happens infrequently, it indicates a high sensitivity to Lomatium Root and this compound should not be used.

COMPOUNDED MELISSA
A Children's Hyperactivity Compound

Contents: Fresh Lemon Balm (Melissa officinalis), Fresh Chamomile Flowers (Matricaria chamomilla), Fresh Passionflower (Passiflora incarnata), Fresh Skullcap Herb (Scutellaria lateriflora), Fresh Wild Oat Seed (Avena sativa), Fresh Gotu Kola Glycerite (Centella asiatica), Mineral salts extracted from Kelp, Irish Moss, and other seaweeds.

Therapeutic Actions: This compound contains nervine and tonic principles which both relax and restore to balance the functions of the brain and nerve cells. Although this compound does not promote sleepiness or lethargy, it quiets down the agitation and over-excitability of the nervous system.

Indications: This compound is very effective in the treatment of children's hyperactivity and anxiety–tetanic patterns, nervous sensitivity and excitability, and attention deficit disorders. As a restorative tonic, this compound may be used during the daytime to reduce hyperactivity and at bedtime to promote deep and efficient sleep. This compound may also be used by adults who exhibit similar difficulties as well as excessive mental chatter and nervous and mental irritation.

Complementary Compounds: To improve the effectiveness of this compound, Compounded Elixir of Passionflower and California Poppy may be used as well as Glycine amino acid.

Uses/Dosage: Add 20–30 drops of extract to a small amount of warm water and take 3–4 times daily between meals. For best results, take this compound for 3–4 months or longer.

COMPOUNDED MILK THISTLE/YELLOW DOCK
A Skin Corrective Compound

Contents: Milk Thistle Seed (Silybum marianum), Fresh Yellow Dock Root (Rumex crispus), Fresh Burdock Root (Arctium lappa), Fresh Echinacea (Echinacea spp.), Sarsaparilla Root (Smilax officinalis), Fresh Oregon Grape Root (Berberis aquafolium).

Therapeutic Actions: This compound targets the organs of metabolism and corrects metabolic errors which are responsible for the manifestation of skin disorders. Yellow Dock addresses skin disorders associated with improper fatty metabolism; Burdock Root addresses skin disorders associated with impure blood; Echinacea addresses skin disorders associated with bacterial growth; Sarsaparilla Root addresses skin disorders associated with hormonal imbalance; and Milk Thistle Seed and Oregon Grape Root addresses skin disorders associated with improper liver metabolism.

Indications: This compound is specifically indicated for a broad spectrum of dermatological conditions including oily acne, cystic acne, hormonal acne, blackheads, pimples, eczema, psoriasis, seborrhea, psoriatic arthritis, and many other skin disturbances. This compound may also be used as a wonderful spring tonic to promote an alteration of catabolic wastes which have built up over the winter. The chemistry and nutrients of the herbs in this compound promote restoration and well-being of the skin as an organ.

Complementary Compounds: This compound may be used compatibly with Compounded Juniper Berry and plenty of warm water throughout the day.

Uses/Dosage: Add 30–40 drops of extract to a small amount of warm water and take 3–4 times daily. Best results are achieved if taken over 3–4 months consecutively.

Contra-indications and Cautions: Do not use this compound during pregnancy.

COMPOUNDED PLANTAIN/BUCHU
A Urinary Incontinence Compound

Contents: Fresh Plantain Leaf and Corm (Plantago lanceolata), African Buchu Leaves (Barosma betulina), Fresh Corn Silk (Zea mays), Fresh Horsetail Grass (Equisetum arvense), Fresh St. John's Wort Flower Buds (Hypericum perforatum), Fresh Arnica Flowers (Arnica latifolia), Fresh Thuja Leaf (Thuja occidentalis).

Therapeutic Actions: The herbs in this compound act to strengthen the musculature and tone the membranes of the urinary system. The soothing and restorative properties of these herbs relieve irritation and weakness of the urinary tract.

Indications: This compound is specifically indicated for urinary incontinence in both children and adults. Also may be used as a restorative tonic to strengthen the musculature of the pelvic organs.

Uses/Dosage: Add 20–30 drops of extract to a small amount of warm water and take 3–4 times daily for up to 2–3 months. Children's dose should be lowered to 5–15 drops 3–4 times daily and taken for 1–2 months.

Contra-indications and Cautions: This compound should not be taken during pregnancy.

COMPOUNDED RED CLOVER
A Blood & Lymphatic Alterative Compound

Contents: Fresh Red Clover Blossoms (Trifolium pratense), Fresh Stinging Nettle Leaf (Urtica dioica), Fresh Cleavers Herb (Galium aparine), Fresh Yellow Dock Root (Rumex crispus), Fresh Burdock Root (Arctium lappa), Fresh Yarrow Flowers (Achillea millefolium), Fresh Plantain Leaf & Corm (Plantago lanceolata), Licorice Root (Glycyrrhiza glabra), Prickly Ash Bark (Xanthoxylum clavaherculis).

Therapeutic Actions: The herbs in this compound are classic blood and lymphatic alteratives which alter the catabolic tissue conditions and bring about an improved state of well-being through improved metabolism and elimination. These herbs target the organs of metabolism, improving their functions and restoring their vitality by carrying more blood and nutrient supply to the cellular level and promoting greater excretion at the cellular level.

Indications: This compound cools excess heat in the blood and liver and may be used specifically in the treatment of cancer, eczema, psoriasis, tumors, cysts, toxemia, lymphedema, swollen and caseated lymph nodes, psoriatic and gouty arthritis, acne, and all skin disturbances. This compound may also be used as a spring tonic to promote detoxification.

Complementary Compounds: This compound combines well with Compounded Juniper Berry and should be used with plenty of warm water throughout the day. (For specific indications please refer to the Herbal Repertory).

Uses/Dosage: Add 30–40 drops of extract to a small amount of warm water and take 3–4 times daily. Best results are achieved if taken for 2–4 months consecutively.

Contra-indications and Cautions: Do not use this compound during pregnancy.

COMPOUNDED ROBERTS FORMULA
A Digestive Corrective Formula

Contents: Fresh Compounded Echinacea (Echinacea angustifolia and Echinacea purpurea), Fresh Marshmallow Root (Althaea officinalis), Fresh Goldenseal Root (Hydrastis canadensis), Fresh Geranium Root (Geranium maculatum), Fresh Slippery Elm Bark (Ulmus rubra), Fresh Poke Root (Phytolacca americana).

Therapeutic Actions: This compound targets the lining of the GI tract and corrects enteric bacterial imbalances and functional disturbances of the entire intestinal tract.

Indications: Useful in the treatment of gastric ulcers, gastric itrritation, irritable bowel syndrome, spastic colon, bacterial imbalances of the colon, toxemia, and digestive metabolic disorders.

Complementary Compounds: If treating gastric ulcers, this compound is most effective if used with Deglycyrrhizinaed Licorice Powder. Also useful to use with Compounded Glyconda Cordial.

Uses/Dosage:	Take 30–50 drops of extract in a small amount of warm water 3–4 times daily between meals.
Contra-indications and Cautions:	Do not use this compound during pregnancy.

COMPOUNDED SAW PALMETTO
A Men's Prostate Compound

Contents:	Fresh Saw Palmetto Berry (Serenoa repens), Fresh Echinacea (Echinacea spp.), Fresh Stinging Nettle Root (Urtica dioica), Poplar Bark (Populus tremulodies), Fresh Pipsissewa Herb (Chimaphila umbellata), Fresh Thuja Leaf (Thuja occidentalis).
Therapeutic Actions:	The herbs in this compound target the prostate gland and surrounding tissues and promote better secretions, better lymphatic drainage, and waste excretions from the genito-urinary system.
Indications:	This compound is indicated in the treatment of benign prostatic hyperplasia (BPH), prostatic infections, prostatitis, gravel, sedimentation, spermatorrhea, difficulty in passing urine freely, nocturnal urination, painful urination.
Complementary Compounds:	For the above-cited conditions, use with Pygeum Bark and Fresh Poke Root extract as well as Compounded Juniper Berry.
Uses/Dosage:	Add 30–50 drops of extract to a small amount of warm water and take 3–4 times daily as a corrective measure. Drink plenty of warm water throughout the day when using this compound.
Contra-indications and Cautions:	If prostatic problems are present, please seek professional naturopathic advice.

COMPOUNDED SCUDDER'S ALTERATIVE
A Deep-Tissue Cleansing Compound

Contents: Corydalis Tubers (Dicentra canadensis), Fresh Black Alder Bark (Alnus serrulata), Mayapple Root (Podophyllum pelatum), Figwort Flowering Herb (Scrophularia nodosa), Fresh Yellow Dock Root (Rumex crispus).

Therapeutic Actions: This excellent alterative compound was originally prepared according to Prof. Scudder's formula (an eclectic medical formula). It acts, as all alteratives do, to replace catabolic tissue with healthy, more vibrant tissue. This is an alterative second to none, working to bring about a repair to the vital force through the removal of obstructing waste material.

Indications: Specifically indicated in liver and glandular afflictions, skin disorders, lymphatic and blood disorders, tumors, cysts, boils, carbuncles, cancers, endometriosis, and conditions where there is waste build-up and deranged tissue.

Complementary Compounds: This compound may be used harmoniously with Compounded Juniper Berry and plenty of warm water.

Uses/Dosage: Add 30–40 drops of extract to a small amount of warm water and take 3–4 times daily. Best results are achieved if taken for 2–4 months consecutively.

Contra-indications and Cautions: Do not use this compound during pregnancy.

COMPOUNDED SHEEP SORREL/BURDOCK
An Alterative Compound for Degenerative Processes

Contents: Fresh Sheep Sorrel (Rumex acetosella), Fresh Burdock Root (Arctium lappa), Fresh Slippery Elm Bark (Ulmus rubra), Turkey Rhubarb Root (Rhuem palmatum).

Therapeutic Actions: This compound is a replication of Renée Caisse's formula used extensively for the treatment of degenerative disorders. It alters the process of waste and nutrition helping to break down catabolic tissue and promote the replacement of wasted tissue with healthy new tissue.

Indications: Use this compound when there is chronic degen-erative illness as a profilactic treatment. May also be used as another fine alterative to aid in the maintenance of a healthy constitution.

Uses/Dosage: Take 30–50 drops of extract in a small amount of warm water and take 3–4 times daily between meals.

**Contra-indications
and Cautions:** Do not take this compound during pregnancy.

 COMPOUNDED SKULLCAP/ST. JOHN'S WORT
A Nerve, Trauma, & Sleep Compound

Contents: Fresh Skullcap Herb (Scutellaria lateriflora), Fresh St. John's Wort Flower Buds (Hypericum perfora-tum), Fresh Calendula Flowers (Calendula offici-nalis), Fresh Chamomile Flowers (Matricaria chamomilla), Fresh California Poppy (Escholzia californica), Fresh Wild Oats (Avena sativa), Fresh Valerian Root (Valeriana officinalis).

Therapeutic Actions: This compound is a nerve restorative, anti-spasmodic, and soothing anodyne formula. The specific herbs in this compound repair damaged and irritated nerves, sooth nervous agitation and excitability, and exert a mild sedative action to help promote sleep.

Indications: This compound is specifically indicated for the treatment of nerve and muscle spasms, nerve trauma, nerve injury, and nervous agitation. As a restorative, it repairs the vital force after injury, trauma, or shock. It is specifically useful in the treatment of anxiety, insomnia, hyper-excitability, tension, nerve exhaustion, and nerve disturbances. This compound can also be used as an anti-viral agent both topically and internally for the treatment of shingles and herpes.

Complementary Compounds:

The actions of the herbs in this compound are enhanced with the use of Compounded Elixir of Passionflower.

Uses/Dosage:

Add 30–40 drops of extract to a small amount of warm water and take 3–4 times daily between meals.

Contra-indications and Cautions:

Do not use this compound during pregnancy.

COMPOUNDED SMILAX/DAMIANA
A Male/Female Virility Compound

Contents:

Sarsaparilla Root (Smilax officinalis), Damiana Herb (Turnera diffusa), Fresh Wild American Ginseng Root (Panax quinquifolium), Ashwaghanda (Winter Cherry—Withenia somnifera), Shatavari Root (Asparagus Root—Asparagus racemosus), Fresh Wild Oat Seed (Avena sativa), Licorice Root (Glycyrrhiza glabra), Hawthorn Berry (Crataegus oxycantha), Prickly Ash Bark (Xanthoxylum clava-herculis).

Therapeutic Actions:

This compound contains natural phytosterols and other natural hormonal like compounds which target the same receptors as endogenous hormones. The herbs bring a natural enlivening influence throughout the body and mind. The restorative and tonic actions of the herbs enable more stamina, vitality, endurance, and virility to be enjoyed.

Indications:

This compound is specifically indicated for individuals desiring greater stamina and virility. It is useful to use as an adjunct to body-building programs and programs designed to enhance athletic performance. It is also useful when there is deficiency and anemia associated with a weak constitution.

**Complementary
Compounds:**

This compound may be used compatibly with Siberian Ginseng Tonic and Compounded Ginseng/Schizandra.

Uses/Dosage:

Add 30–40 drops of extract to a small amount of warm water and take 3–4 times daily between meals. Best results are achieved if taken over a 3–4 month period.

**Contra-indications
and Cautions:**

Do not take this compound during pregnancy.

COMPOUNDED SPILANTHES
An Anti-Yeast & Anti-Fungal Compound

Contents:

Fresh Spilanthes Flowering Tops & Root (Spilanthes acmella), Fresh Oregon Grape Root (Berberis aquafolium), Fresh Juniper Berry (Junipers communis), Usnea Lichen (Usnea spp.), Myrrh Gum (Commiphora molmol).

Therapeutic Actions:

The herbs in this compound contain natural anti-fungal, antibacterial, and anti-yeast properties.

Indications:

This compound is specifically indicated in the treatment of Candida Yeast overgrowth, vaginal infections, fungal infections (finger and toenail fungus), athlete's foot, and ringworm. This compound may also be used as an adjunct in the treatment of Epstein Barr Virus (EBV).

**Complementary
Compounds:**

The use of Compounded Elixir of Bitters is very effective as an adjunct to overcoming yeast overgrowth.

Uses/Dosage:

Add 30–40 drops of extract to a small amount of

warm water and take 3–4 times daily between meals. Best results are achieved if taken over a period of 3–4 months.

Contra-indications and Cautions:

Do not take this compound during pregnancy.

COMPOUNDED TURMERIC/CATECHU
An Immediate-Type Hypersensitivity/Allergy & Anti-Inflammatory Compound

Contents:

Fresh Turmeric Root (Curcuma longa), Black Catechu (Catechu nigra), Fresh Grindelia Floral Buds (Grindelia robusta), Licorice Root (Glycyrrhiza glabra), Rose Hips (Rosa rugosa), Chinese Skullcap (Scutellaria baicalensis), Fresh Ginkgo Leaf (Ginkgo biloba), African Devil's Claw Root (Harpagophytum procumbens), Fresh Yarrow Flowers (Achellia millefolium), Fresh Lobelia Herb & Seed (Lobelia inflata).

Therapeutic Actions:

The herbs in this compound contain active constituents which act as anti-inflammatory, anti-histamine, bronchial dilators, respiratory anti-spasmodics, and membrane integrity enhancers. Also, these herbs are powerful anti-hepato-toxic in that they protect the liver from circulating anti-gens/allergens. This compound is formulated to provide adrenal support when epinephrine is needed by the body to compensate for the inflam-matory responses generated from the presence of allergens. A specific mode of action of this com-pound is to stabilize mast cells of the respiratory membranes, mucous membranes, and epidermal skin tissue.

Indications:

This compound is specifically indicated for the treatment of all disorders of immediate-type hyper-sensitivity including allergies, asthma, urticaria, reactive dermatitis, reactive arthritis, reactive irritable bowel syndrome, anaphylaxis, food sensitivities,

43

sinusitis, and other acute and chronic inflammations.

Complementary Compounds: As an adjunct to the therapy please refer to other formulas listed in this section as well as in the Herbal Repertory section. Specifically, refer to the pull-out section at the end of the book entitled "Botanical Protocols for Disorders of Immediate-Type Hypersensitivity."

Uses/Dosage: Add 30–40 drops of extract to a small amount of warm water and take 4–5 times daily between meals. Best results are achieved if taken for 3–4 months. Drink plenty of warm water while using this compound.

COMPOUNDED USNEA/UVA URSI
A Urinary Tract Antibiotic Formula

Contents: Usnea Lichen (Usnea spp.), Fresh Uva Ursi Leaf (Arctostaphylos uva ursi), Fresh Pipsissewa Leaf (Chimaphila umbellata), Fresh Echinacea (Echinacea spp.).

Therapeutic Actions: This compound contains natural antibiotic and antibacterial compounds which target directly the urinary system.

Indications: This compound is specifically indicated in the treatment of bladder infections, kidney infections, urinary tract infections, and cystitis, as well as nephritis. This preparation may also be used for chronic urinary irritation and chronic bladder irritation.

Complementary Compounds: Add to the above compound Uva Ursi Solid Extract.

Uses/Dosage: Add 40–60 drops of extract to a small amount of warm water and take every 1–2 hours until symptoms of urinary infections disappear. Use this formula for a maximum of 5–7 days only.

Contra-indications and Cautions: Do not use this compound during pregnancy. Use only for a maximum of 5–7 days. If symptoms of urinary tract infections are present, please consult your naturopathic physician. Do not use this formula with cranberry juice as the juice will neutralize the actions of the herbs.

COMPOUNDED VITEX/ALFALFA
A Menopausal Corrective Compound

Contents: Chaste Tree Berry (Vitex agnus-castus), Alfalfa Leaf (Medicago sativa), Night Blooming Cereus (Cactus grandiflorus), St. John's Wort Flower Buds (Hypericum perforatum), Sage Leaf (Salvia officinalis), Fresh Wild Oat Seed (Avena sativa), Fresh Motherwort Flowering Tops (Leonurus cardiaca), Essential Oil of Lavender.

Therapeutic Actions: The herbs in this compound assist in the balancing of the Follicle Stimulating Hormone (F.S.H.) and the Luteal Hormone (L.H.). This compound has a restorative effect upon the corpus luteum and enables the body to maintain a minimal amount of progesterone secretion from the corpus luteum which in turn enables estrogen levels to increase. Also, this compound addresses symptoms which are prevalent during menopause. These symptoms normalize as the hormones become balanced.

Indications: This compound is specifically indicated for the treatment of hot flashes, night sweats, depression, skin changes and anxiety during menopause, and other changes such as bone loss (osteoporosis) during menopause.

Complementary Compounds: This compound should be used with Compounded Elixir of Vitex and Alfalfa Solid Extract and Wild Yam Extract as natural substitutes for estrogen replacement therapy.

Uses/Dosage: Add 30–40 drops of extract to a small amount of warm water and take 3–4 times daily between meals. Best results are achieved if taken for 3–4 months consecutively.

COMPOUNDED WILD CHERRY
An Anti-Coughing Compound

Contents: Fresh Wild Cherry Bark (Prunus serotina), Fresh Elecampane Root (Inula helenium), Yerba Santa Leaf (Eriodictyon californicum), Fresh Red Clover Blossoms (Trifolium pratense), Licorice Root (Glycyrrhiza glabra), Fresh Butterbur Root (Petasites frigida).

Therapeutic Actions: This compound contains respiratory antispasmodic principles and soothing emollient principles which target the lungs and respiratory membranes.

Indications: This compound is used in the treatment of dry, irritative coughs, whooping cough, asthmatic cough, spastic cough, bronchial irritation. It loosens hardened catarrh from the respiratory lining and promotes the expectoration of this catarrh and mucous.

Complementary Compounds: This compound may be used with any of the following herbs in the treatment of spastic coughs: Lobelia, Grindelia, Marshmallow Root, Comfrey Root, Slippery Elm Bark, Pleurisy Root, and Lungwort Lichen.

Dosage: Add 30–50 drops of extract to a small amount of warm water and take 3–5 times daily between meals. Use as often as necessary to relieve the symptoms of irritative cough.

COMPOUNDED YUCCA/BURDOCK
An Anti-Arthritic/Anti-Inflammatory Compound

Contents: Fresh Yucca Root (Yucca spp.), Fresh Echinacea (Echinacea spp.), Fresh Burdock Root & Seed

(Arctium lappa), Fresh Poke Root (Phytolacca americana), Celery Seed (Apium graveolens), Bladderwrack Fronds (Fucus versiculosis), Fresh Pipsissewa Herb (Chimaphilla umbellata).

Therapeutic Actions: The herbs in this compound have strong anti-inflammatory compounds. Specific actions also include diuretic properties as well as properties to alkalize an over-acid body chemistry which is generally associated with arthritis.

Indications: This compound is indicated for the treatment of gouty arthritis, psoriatic arthritis, articular rheumatism (rheumatism of the small joints), and arthritis associated with a febrile constitution (over-acid body chemistry). The herbs in this compound dislodge acids and crystals in tissues and promote their excretion through the urinary system.

Complementary Compounds: This compound should be used with Compounded Red Clover and Compounded Juniper Berry to accent the effectiveness of the herbs. Use plenty of warm water when taking this compound.

Dosage: Add 30–40 drops of extract to a small amount of warm water and take 3–5 times daily between meals. Best results are achieved if taken over 3–4 months consecutively.

Contra-indications and Cautions: Do not use this compound during pregnancy.

FRESH PLANT ELIXIRS
Rejuvenative Tonics

The compounds listed below are best prepared and used as herbal elixirs. In this fashion they are truly tonic to the physiology and rejuvenate the deep body tissues of the systems which they target. One of the key features of these Elixir Compounds is the addition of several species of sea vegetation and marine algae to the formulation. The micro-nutrition contained within the seaweeds provides a rich source of minerals and trace minerals which target the same receptors the primary herbs in the compound target. In this way, the tissues and cells of the body not only receive the influence of the plants, but also the influence of the micro-nutrition. Thus, the vital force is fortified at the tissue and cellular level. The end result is a very deep restoration and rejuvenation of the organs and systems which the Elixir Compounds target.

COMPOUNDED REJUVENATIVE ELIXIR

Contents: Amalaki (Indian Gooseberry), Siberian Ginseng, Fresh Gotu Kola Leaf and Root, Fresh Ginkgo Leaf, Fresh Ligustrum Berry, Prickly Ash Bark, Hawthorn Berry Solid Extract, Rose Hip Solid Extract, Concentrated Apricot and Mulberry Syrup, Custom Extract of Sea Vegetation and Marine Algae, Vegetable Glycerine.

Actions & Indications: Promotes longevity of body tissues, balances the composition of the blood and lymph and regenerates healthy brain and nerve cells. Supports the immune system and enhances energy and clarity of perception. Use specifically as a tonic to renew the vitality of the body and mind.

Dosage: Use 1 teaspoon 3 times daily between meals.

COMPOUNDED VITAMIN C ELIXIR

Contents: Amalaki (Indian Gooseberry), Rose Hips Solid Extract, Custom Extract of Sea Vegetation and Marine Algae, Sweet Orange Essence, Vegetable Glycerine.

Actions & Indications: Use as an organic plant source of Vitamin C. Derived from Amalaki fruits growing wild in India, each fruit contains nearly 3,000 mg of organic Vitamin C. The actions of this delicious elixir are: to strongly enhance body immune response against colds, flus, and infections; to enhance capillary integrity; to rebuild and maintain body tissues; and to enhance the vitality of every cell.

Dosage: Use 1 teaspoon 3 times daily between meals.

COMPOUNDED NUTRITIONAL ELIXIR

Contents: Fresh Nettle Leaf, Fresh Wild Oats, Fresh Red Clover Blossoms, Fresh Red Raspberry Leaf, Fresh Yellow Dock Roots, Fresh Gentian Roots, Fresh Elderberries, Amalaki (Indian Gooseberry), Alfalfa Solid Extract, Rose Hips Solid Extract, Hawthorn Berry Solid Extract, Concentrated Syrup of Apricots & Mulberries, Chlorella, Custom Extract of Sea Vegetation and Marine Algae, Vegetable Glycerine.

Actions & Indications: The rich mineral salts represented in this compounded tonic invigorate the blood chemistry and normalize iron deficiency, enabling more vital oxygen to nourish the brain cells. A specific for anemics or any deficiency or as an alterative to any vitamin/mineral supplement. Can also be used as an energy tonic providing more vitality to body and mind. This compound also facilitates and enhances enzyme activity promoting an increased uptake of nutrition into the cells.

Dosage: Use 1 teaspoon 3 times daily between meals.

COMPOUNDED CALCIUM ELIXIR

Contents: Fresh Comfrey Root, Fresh Marshmallow Root, Fresh Black Walnut Leaf & Hulls, Fresh Skullcap Herb, Fresh Mullein Leaf, Fresh St. John's Wort Flower Buds, Fresh White Oak Bark, Fresh Gravel Root, Fresh Horsetail Herb, Hawthorn Berry Solid Extract, Mineral Ash of Alfalfa Leaf and Nettle Leaf, Concentrated Extract of Sea Vegetation and Marine Algae (especially Kelp and Bladderwrack).

Actions & Indications: A Bone, Flesh, Cartilage and Connective Tissue Formula. Use as an agent to facilitate the uptake of calcium salt and to promote the healing of wounds, injuries, broken bones, burns, torn cartilage, torn ligaments, etc. Also very effective in promoting quick recovery after a chronic illness by strengthening the vital force.

Dosage: 1 teaspoon 3–4 times daily when needed. Use for up to 3 months consecutively then discontinue its use for 2–3 months.

COMPOUNDED ELIXIR OF PASSIONFLOWER

Contents: Fresh Passionflower, Fresh Skullcap Herb, Fresh Chamomile Flowers, Fresh Hops Strobile, Fresh Wild Oats, Fresh Mugwort Leaf, Fresh Peppermint Leaf, Hawthorn Berry Solid Extract, Concentrated Apricot & Mulberry Syrup, Custom Extract of Sea Vegetation and Marine Algae, Vegetable Glycerine, Peppermint Essence.

Actions & Indications: A Nerve Tonic and Restorative. Especially useful in anxiety conditions, hyperactivity, trauma, restlessness, and insomnia. The elixir fortifies the nerve cells with rich trace elements, enhances nerve vitality, relieves tissue tension in the stomach and digestive tract, and encourages a free flow of nerve energy through the physiology. This is not a sedative and can be used during the daytime to counteract anxiety, and at night to facilitate easy sleep.

Dosage: Use 1 teaspoon 3 times daily between meals.

COMPOUNDED ELIXIR OF SIBERIAN GINSENG

Contents: Siberian Ginseng Solid Extract, Royal Jelly, Schizandra Berries, Fresh Yellow Dock Root, Fresh Gentian Root, Prickly Ash Bark, Rose Hips Solid Extract, Chlorella, Custom Extract of Sea Vegetation and Marine Algae.

Actions & Indications: An adaptogenic tonic useful in all deficient constitutions. Useful as an adjunct in building blood and raising the quality of the vital force. Provides increased energy, strength and clarity. Excellent tonic for rehabilitation and geriatrics. A specific for anemia, deficient menses, physical weakness of long standing nature and immune deficient syndromes.

Dosage: $1/2$–1 teaspoon 3 times daily between meals.

COMPOUNDED ELIXIR OF BITTERS

Contents: Amalaki (Indian Gooseberry), Fresh Turmeric Root, Mature Milk Thistle Seed, Fresh Wild Yam Root, Fennel Seed, Cardamon Seed, Fresh Calamus Root, Anise Seed, Bitter Orange Oil, Ginger Root, Custom Extract of Sea Vegetation and Marine Algae.

Actions & Indications: A Sweet/Bitter Digestive Tonic. An extremely valuable aid in revitalizing the digestive functions by enhancing secretions of the liver, pancreas, stomach, and small intestine. This compounded elixir provides rich enzyme catalysts which improve nutrient absorption. This compound also protects the liver from endogenous toxins and normalizes gut and intestinal flora. Other indications include flatulence, constipation, abdominal bloating, digestive distress, and sluggish peristalsis.

Dosage: Use $1/2$ teaspoon in warm water 3 times daily before meals.

COMPOUNDED ELIXIR OF VITEX

Contents: Fresh Chaste Tree Berry, Fresh Squaw Vine, Fresh Black Haw Bark, Fresh Butterbur Root, Fresh Mugwort Leaf, Fresh Dandelion Leaf and Root,

Usnea Lichen, Rose Hips Solid Extract, Concentrated Mulberry Syrup, Custom Extract of Sea Vegetation and Marine Algae, Vegetable Glycerine.

Actions & Indications:

A Female Hormonal Corrective Formula. This compounded elixir corrects imbalances of estrogen metabolism associated with excessive catachol-estrogens and elevated inflammatory prostaglandins. Therefore, it is very useful in the treatment of PMS syndrome, amenorrhea, dysmenorrhea, endometriosis, and menopausal imbalances.

Dosage:

Use 1 teaspoon 3 times daily between meals. This compounded elixir must be used for 4–6 months consecutively. During the pre-menstrual phase, dosage may be increased to 1 teaspoon 4–5 times daily.

COMPOUNDED ELIXIR OF ELEUTHEROX

Contents:

Siberian Ginseng, Sarsaparilla Root Solid Extract, Fresh Saw Palmetto Berry, Fresh Ligustrum Berry, Rose Hips Solid Extract, Fresh Dandelion Root and Leaf, Usnea Lichen, Concentrated Mulberry Syrup, Custom Extract of Sea Vegetation and Marine Algae, Vegetable Glycerine.

Actions & Indications:

A Male Revitalizing Tonic. Useful for athletes during workout phase, for energy enhancement, and increased physical endurance. This compound may provide steroidal-like activity, thus its value in athletic training.

Dosage:

Use 1 teaspoon 3 times daily between meals.

Index To The Herbal Repertory: Botanical Treatment Protocols

This clinical repertory is divided into the major body systems. Major imbalances are listed within each system with proper botanical treatments. This repertory provides an opportunity for the reader to become acquainted with a more clinical approach to medical herbalism. This section in no way supports an allopathic model of herbal usage. It is not intended to provide the reader with diagnostic or prescriptive advice for the treatment of specific illnesses. This information is solely for educational purposes. The remedies given are the collected information of materia medicas, U.S. Dispensatorics, and clinical repertories as well as the author's clinical experience. The reader should consult a fully licensed naturopathic physician for any medical condition present. This herbal repertory is not intended as a substitute for medical care.

BLOOD AND LYMPHATIC SYSTEM
Herbal Agents Influencing the Blood and Lymph

ANEMIA
Compounded Nutritional Elixir, Yellow Dock Root, Chlorella, Alfalfa Solid extract

BLOOD CLOTS
Melilot Herb, Compounded Red Clover, Prickly Ash Bark, Compounded Echinacea/Red Root, Compounded Scudder's Alterative, Hawthorn

BLOOD DYSCRASIA
Fresh Baptisia Root, Compounded Echinacea/Red Root, Fresh Thuja Leaf, Compounded Scudder's Alterative

BLOOD POISONING
Compounded Echinacea, Lobelia Herb & Seed

CANCER

Compounded Hoxsey/Red Clover, Compounded Echinacea/Red Root, Fresh Thuja Leaf, Astragalus Root, Fresh Yellow Dock Root, Compounded Sheep Sorrel/Burdock

To the above add the following specifics:

Brain Cancer

Mistletoe Extract, Chaparral Extract, Venus' Flytrap Extract

Breast Cancer

Fresh Goldenseal Root, Fresh Poke Root, Compounded Echinacea, Fresh Blue Flag Root, Venus' Flytrap Extract

Colon/Liver/Pancreas Cancer

Chaparral Leaf, Turmeric Root Extract, Bromalain, Venus' Flytrap Extract

Kidney Cancer

Mistletoe Extract, Turmeric Root Extract, Bromalain, Venus' Flytrap Extract

Lung Cancer

Mistletoe Extract, Turmeric Root Extract, Fresh Poke Root, Bromalain, Venus' Flytrap Extract

Prostate Cancer

Fresh Saw Palmetto Berry, Mistletoe Extract, Fresh Poke Root, Turmeric Root Extract, Bromalain

Stomach Cancer

Turmeric Root Extract, Bromalain, Venus' Flytrap Extract

Uterine/Ovarian Cancer

Turmeric Root Extract, Bromalain, Fresh Poke Root Extract, Venus' Flytrap Extract

CASEATED LYMPH NODES

Compounded Echinacea/Red Root, Fresh Poke Root Extract, Fresh Baptisia Root, Compounded Hoxsey/Red Clover,

Goldenseal Root, Compounded Mullein/ Lobelia Salve topically.

Hodgkin's Disease
Madagascar Periwinkle, Compounded Hoxsey/ Red Clover, Mistletoe Extract, Compounded Echinacea/Red Root, Turmeric Root Extract, Bromalain, Venus' Flytrap Extract

Leukemia
Compounded Echinacea/Red Root, Compounded Hoxsey/ Red Clover, Fresh Baptisia Root, Fresh Thuja leaf

LYMPHATIC ENGORGEMENT
Compounded Echinacea/Red Root, Fresh Thuja Leaf, Fresh Baptisia Root, Compounded Red Clover, Compounded Juniper Berry, Fresh Poke Root

LYMPHATIC SWELLING
Compounded Echinacea/Red Root, Fresh Poke Root, Compounded Mullein/Lobelia Salve topically

LYMPHEDEMA
Fresh Cleavers Herb, Compounded Red Clover, Compounded Juniper Berry

MASTITIS
Compounded Mullein/Lobelia Salve (topically), Thuja Oil (topically), Fresh Thuja Leaf, Compounded Echinacea/Red Root, Fresh Poke Root Oil (Topically), Fresh Poke Root

CARDIOVASCULAR SYSTEM
Herbal Agents Influencing the Heart and Coronary Vascular System

★Use only with physician's care.

ARRYTHMIAS
Hawthorn Berry Solid Extract, Compounded Hawthorn, Fresh Motherwort Extract, Lily of the Valley★, Cactus Grandiflorus Extract

ARTERIOSCLEROSIS
Hawthorn Berry Solid Extract, Compounded Hawthorn, Bladderwrack Extract, Compounded Calcium Elixir

ANGINA PECTORIS
Hawthorn Berry Solid Extract, Compounded
Hawthorn, Cactus Grandiflorus Extract

CARDIAC IRRITABILITY
Compounded Bugleweed/Motherwort, Compounded Hawthorn, Cactus Grandiflorus Extract

CONGESTIVE HEART FAILURE
Cactus Grandiflorus Extract, Compounded Hawthorn

HYPERTENSION
Compounded Linden/Crataegus, Hawthorn Berry
Solid Extract, Compounded Hawthorn, Valerian
Root, Wild Oats, Siberian Ginseng Root,
Rauwolfia Root Extract

HYPOTENSION
Siberian Ginseng Root, Fresh Wild Oats, Hawthorn
Berry Solid Extract, Cactus Grandiflorus Extract

MITRAL VALVE INSUFFICIENCY
Hawthorn Berry Solid Extract, Cactus Grandiflorus Extract, Lily of the Valley★

NERVOUS HEART
Compounded Hawthorn, Compounded Bugleweed/Motherwort, Compounded Calcium Elixir

CARDIAC PALPITATIONS
Compounded Bugleweed/Motherwort,
Compounded Hawthorn

PERICARDITIS
Hawthorn Berry Solid Extract, Lily of the Valley★

TACHYCARDIA
Compounded Bugleweed/Motherwort,
Compounded Hawthorn

★*Use only with physician's care.*

DIGESTIVE SYSTEM
Herbal Agents Influencing
the Digestive Functions

ABDOMINAL PAIN
With pressure on pelvic viscera
Fringe Tree, Life Root, Fresh Helonias Root, Fresh
Chaste Tree, Compounded Fraxinus/Ceanothus

CIRRHOSIS
Fringe Tree, Schizandra Berry, Milk Thistle Seed,
Eclipta alba, Phyllanthus amarus

DYSPEPSIA
Compounded Elixir of Bitters, Glyconda
Neutralizing Cordial

GALL STONES
Dandelion Root and Leaf, Compounded Dande-
lion/Fennel, Bladderwrack Extract, Fresh Gravel
Root Extract, Compounded Fennel/Wild Yam

GASTRITIS
Fresh Gentian Root, Fennel Seed, Compounded
Elixir of Bitters, Glyconda Neutralizing Cordial

HEPATITIS
Milk Thistle Seed, Fringe Tree, Schizandra Berry,
Eclipta alba, Phyllanthus amarus

INDIGESTION
Compounded Elixir of Bitters, Compounded
Dandelion/Fennel, Glyconda Neutralizing Cordial

JAUNDICE
Fringe Tree

PAIN
Right-sided
Fresh Celandine Root and Tops, Compounded
Elixir of Bitters, Dandelion Root, Glyconda
Neutralizing Cordial
Left-sided
Milk Thistle Seed, Red Root, Compounded Elixir
of Bitters, Glyconda Neutralizing Cordial

**ENDOCRINE
(GLANDULAR) SYSTEM**
Herbal Agents Influencing
the Glandular Functions

PANCREATITIS
Turmeric Root Extract, Compounded Elixir of
Bitters, Fringe Tree

ADRENAL GLANDS

Adrenal Insufficiency
Fresh Wild Oats, Licorice Root, Siberian Ginseng,
Fo-Ti Extract, Compounded Elixir of Siberian
Ginseng, Compounded Ginseng/Schizandra

Adrenal Exhaustion
With cardiac arrythmias
Cactus Grandiflorus Extract, Compounded
Hawthorn

LYMPHATICS
See listing under Blood and Lymphatic System

MAMMARY GLANDS

Cancer
Compounded Hoxsey/Red Clover, Com-
pounded Echinacea/Red Root, Fresh Poke
Root, Mistletoe Extract, Chaparral Extract,
Turmeric Root Extract, Bromalain, Venus'
Flytrap, Compounded Sheep Sorrel/Burdock

Fibroids
Fresh Thuja Leaf, Compounded Echinacea/Red
Root, Fresh Poke Root, Fresh Goldenseal Root,
Compounded Mullein/Lobelia Salve topically,
Castor Oil topically, Fresh Poke Root Oil topically

Painful
Compounded Mullein/Lobelia salve topically,
Castor oil topically

PITUITARY GLANDS
Fresh Gotu Kola Leaf and Root, Compounded
Gotu Kola, Chaste Tree Extract

PROSTATE GLAND
See listing under Reproductive System

THYROID GLAND

Goiter
Bladderwrack Extract, Fresh Thuja Leaf, Fresh
Blue Flag Root, Mullein/Lobelia salve topically

Hypoactivity
Bladderwrack Extract

Grave's Disease
Compounded Calcium Elixir, Compounded
Bugleweed/Motherwort, Cactus Grandiflorus,
Compounded Hawthorn

Hyperactivity
Compounded Calcium Elixir, Compounded
Bugleweed/Motherwort, Lemon Balm,
Compounded Melissa

GASTROINTESTINAL SYSTEM
Herbal Agents
Influencing the Colon
and Small Intestine

ABDOMINAL BLOATING
Compounded Elixir of Bitters, Fennel Seed,
Compounded Dandelion/Fennel, Glyconda
Neutralizing Cordial

COLITIS
Marshmallow Root, Licorice Root, Bowel
Cleansing Powder, Roberts' Formula, Slippery Elm

COLITIS
Ulcerative
Bowel Cleansing Powder, Marshmallow Root,
Licorice Root, Goldenseal Root, Compounded
Echinacea, Roberts' Formula, Slippery Elm

CONSTIPATION
With Deficient Glandular Secretions
Fresh Goldenseal Root, Prickly Ash Bark,
Internal Cleansing Program, Compounded
Scudder's Alterative

With Deficient Peristalsis
Bowel Cleansing Powder, Cascara Sagrada Bark,
Compounded Scudder's Alterative
With Flatulence
Butternut Bark, Fennel Seed, Compounded Bitter
Elixir, Glyconda Neutralizing Cordial
With Hardened Feces
Internal Cleansing Program, Celandine Root and
Tops (short term use), Cascara Sagrada Bark,
Compounded Scudder's Alterative

DIARRHEA
With mucous and coldness
Ginger Root, Red Raspberry Leaf, Bayberry
Root Bark, Geranium Root

DIVERTICULITIS
Bowel Cleansing Powder, Marshmallow Root,
Licorice Root, Roberts' Formula

FLATULENCE
Fennel Seed, Compounded Elixir of Bitters

HEMORRHOIDS
Fresh Collinsonia Root, Witch Hazel, Fresh
Goldenseal Root, Marshmallow Root, St. John's
Wort Oil topically, Comfrey Compound Oil
topically

HEMORRHOIDS
Bleeding
Fresh Collinsonia Root, Fresh Goldenseal Root,
Fresh Marshmallow Root, St. John's Wort Oil
topically, Comfrey Compound Oil topically

IRRITABLE BOWEL SYNDROME
Enteric Peppermint oil, Fresh Marshmallow Root,
Bowel Cleansing Powder, Licorice Root, Fresh
Goldenseal Root, Roberts' Formula

MUCOUS MEMBRANE SYSTEM
Herbal Agents
Influencing the Eyes,
Ears, Nose & Throat

EYES

Cataracts
Herbal eyewash with Rue, Greater Celandine, Dusty Miller, Goldenseal Root, and Eyebright

Conjunctivitis
Eyebright, Fresh Thuja Leaf, Chamomile compresses

Catarrhal Drainage
Compounded Eyebright/Bayberry

Pain
Chamomile compresses

Strain
Gelsemium Root★

EARS

Inflammation
Mullein Flower oil drops, Hypericum Flower oil drops

Otitis
Mullein Flower oil drops or Compounded Mullein/Hypericum Oil Drops

Earache
Mullein Flower oil drops

Tinnitus
Fresh Ginkgo Leaf, Compounded Gotu Kola

NOSE

Catarrh
Compounded Eyebright/Bayberry

Sinus Congestion
Compounded Eyebright/Bayberry, Ginger Oil Drops

Hay Fever
Compounded Eyebright/Bayberry, Fresh

★*Use only with physician's care.*

Stinging Nettle leaf, Compounded Echinacea/
Goldenseal, Compounded Turmeric/Catechu

THROAT

Laryngitis
Fresh Collinsonia Root, Fresh Horseradish
Root, Fresh Goldenseal Root

Pharyngitis
Fresh Red Root, Fresh Horseradish Root

Tonsilitis
Compounded Echinacea/Red Root, Compounded Echinacea/Goldenseal, Fresh Thuja Leaf

Sore Throat
Compounded Echinacea, Compounded
Echinacea/Goldenseal (spray on surface tissue),
Fresh Collinsonia Root

MUCOUS MEMBRANES

Catarrh
Compounded Eyebright/Bayberry,
Compounded Echinacea

Infections
Compounded Echinacea, Compounded
Echinacea/Goldenseal

Vaginitis
Compounded Echinacea/Red Root, Fresh
Spilanthes Tops and Root, Compounded
Spilanthes (internally and as douche)

Yeast Infections
Compounded Spilanthes, Compounded
Lomatium

Fungal Infections
Compounded Spilanthes, Fresh Spilanthes Tops
and Root topically, Fresh Black Walnut Leaf
and Hulls

MUSCULO-SKELETAL SYSTEM
Herbal Agents
Influencing the Muscles
and Structure

ARTHRITIS
Compounded Red Clover, Compounded Juniper Berry. To these general remedies add the following specifics:

Articular Rheumatoid Arthritis (Joints)
Compounded Devil's Claw/Chaparral; Compounded Turmeric/Catechu; Fresh Blue Cohosh Root; compound containing the following herbs: Compounded Yucca/Burdock, Compounded Feverfew/Jamaican Dogwood. Use Compounded Essential Oil Salve topically. For analgesic action, use White Willow Bark.

Muscular Rheumatoid Arthritis (Including Fibrocytis/Myocytis)
Compounded Devil's Claw/Chaparral; Compounded Turmeric/Catechu; Fresh Black Cohosh Root; compound containing the following herbs: Compounded Yucca/Burdock, Compounded Feverfew/Jamaican Dogwood. Use Compounded Essential Oil Salve topically.

Gouty Arthritis
Compounded Devil's Claw/Chaparral, Fresh Pipsissewa Herb, Fresh Juniper Berry, Fresh Burdock Root and Seed, Fresh Stinging Nettle Leaf, Prickly Ash Bark, Compounded Yucca/Burdock. Fresh Ginkgo may be added to assist circulation.

Osteoporosis
Liquid Vitamin K, Alfalfa Solid Extract, Compounded Calcium Elixir, Compounded Elixir of Vitex, Fresh Chaste Tree Extract, Bladderwrack Extract, Compounded Nutritional Elixir

INJURIES
Compounded Comfrey Salve or Oil topically, St. John's Wort Oil topically, Arnica and Calendula Flower Oil topically, Compounded Calcium Elixir

MUSCULAR ACHES

Compounded Essential Oil Salve topically, Fresh Black Cohosh Root, Lobelia Herb and Seed, Arnica Oil topically, Skullcap, Valerian Root, Compounded Feverfew/Jamaican Dogwood

ALZHEIMER'S DISEASE

Fresh Ginkgo Leaf, Compounded Gotu Kola, Fresh Turmeric Root, Fresh Passionflower

ANXIETY

Compounded Elixir of Passionflower, Compounded Skullcap/St. John's Wort, Compounded Melissa

ATTENTION DEFICIT DISORDER

Compounded Melissa, Compounded Elixir of Passionflower, Irish Moss, Kelp

DEPRESSION

Fresh St. John's Wort, Fresh Gotu Kola Leaf and Root, Compounded Gotu Kola, Compounded Melissa

EPILEPSY

Fresh Black Cohosh, Fresh Passionflower, Fresh Skullcap, Fresh Lobelia Herb and Seed

HEADACHES

Due to Cold and Flu

Meadowsweet Extract, White Willow Bark Extract, Compounded Feverfew/Jamaican Dogwood

Migraine

Fresh Feverfew Extract, Compounded Feverfew/Jamaican Dogwood, Fresh Ginkgo Leaf

Stress (With Shoulder and Neck Discomfort and Tension)

Fresh Black Haw Bark, Jamaican Dogwood, Fresh

NERVOUS SYSTEM
Herbal Agents
Influencing the
Nerve Functions

Skullcap, Fresh Valerian Root, Compounded Feverfew/Jamaican Dogwood

Digestive
Fresh Hops Strobile, Fresh Lavender, Fresh Chamomile, Fresh Black Haw Bark

HYPERACTIVITY
Compounded Melissa, Compounded Elixir of Passionflower

HYSTERIA
Fresh Skullcap Herb, Compounded Skullcap/St. John's Wort

INSOMNIA
Compounded Elixir of Passionflower, Compounded Skullcap/St. John's Wort, Fresh Hops Strobile, Fresh Valerian Root

MULTIPLE SCLEROSIS
Hawthorn Berry Solid Extract, Concentrated Fresh Wild Oats, Compounded Elixir of Passionflower, Compounded Skullcap/St. John's Wort, Compounded Melissa, Fresh Turmeric Root, Fresh Gotu Kola Leaf and Root

NEURALGIA
Compounded Feverfew/Jamaican Dogwood, Compounded Skullcap/St. John's Wort, Fresh Valerian Root, Meadowsweet Extract, White Willow Bark Extract

SCIATICA
Compounded Skullcap/St. John's Wort, Fresh Valerian Root, Jamaican Dogwood, Meadowsweet Extract

SPASMS
Fresh Black Haw Bark, Fresh Black Cohosh Root,

Jamaican Dogwood, Fresh Lobelia Herb and Seed, Compounded Feverfew/Jamaican Dogwood

TINNITUS
Fresh Ginkgo Leaf, Compounded Gotu Kola.

FEMALE REPRODUCTIVE SYSTEM

Amenorrhea (Absence of Menses)
Compounded Dong Quai, Compounded Elixir of Vitex; see page GYNE 7

Dysmenorrhea (Painful Menstruation)
Compounded Elixir of Vitex, Compounded Dong Quai, Compounded Feverfew/Jamaican Dogwood, Cramp Bark, Black Haw, Jamaican Dogwood; see page GYNE 7

Endometriosis
Compounded Elixir of Vitex, Fresh Chaste Tree Extract, Compounded Dong Quai, Compounded Fraxinus/Ceanothus, Compounded Echinacea/Red Root, Scudder's Alterative; see page GYNE 9

Infertility
Fresh Helonias Root, Fresh Chaste Tree Extract, Chinese Dong Quai Root, Octocossinol; see page GYNE 12

Menopause
Compounded Elixir of Vitex, Fresh Chaste Tree Extract, Alfalfa Solid Extract, Compounded Vitex/Alfalfa; see pages GYNE 9–12

Menorrhagia
(Excessive Menstrual Bleeding)
Compounded Dong Quai, Compounded Elixir of Vitex, Fresh Helonias Root, Compounded Echinacea/Red Root, Fresh Goldenseal Root, Fresh Yarrow Flower Extract, Shepherd's Purse Extract, Wild Yam Extract; see page GYNE 7

Ovarian Cysts
Compounded Fraxinus/Ceanothus, Fresh Poke Root, Fresh Thuja Leaf, Fresh Gelsemium Root★, Scudder's Alterative, Compounded Gelsemium/Phytolacca★; see page GYNE 8

Premenstrual Syndrome (PMS)
Compounded Elixir of Vitex, Compounded Dong Quai, Fresh Helonias Root, Evening Primrose Oil; see pages GYNE 1–6

Uterine Fibroids
Compounded Fraxinus/Ceanothus, Compounded Echinacea/Red Root, Fresh Poke Root, Fresh Black Cohosh root, Fresh Gelsemium Root★, Scudder's Alterative; see page GYNE 8

Vaginitis
Marshmallow Root and Calendula Flower douche, Compounded Spilanthes internally and as douche

MALE REPRODUCTIVE SYSTEM

Benign Prostatic Hypertrophy (BPH)
Compounded Saw Palmetto, Fresh Thuja Leaf, Compounded Juniper Berry

Prostate Infection
Compounded Saw Palmetto, Fresh Thuja Leaf, Compounded Echinacea

Prostatitis
Compounded Saw Palmetto, Fresh Thuja Leaf

RESPIRATORY SYSTEM
Herbal Agents
Influencing the
Respiratory Functions

ASTHMA
Compounded Wild Cherry, Compounded Turmeric/Catechu, Chinese Ephedra Extract, Fresh Comfrey Root, Fresh Mullein Extract, Fresh Lobelia Herb and Seed, Fresh Marshmallow Root, Fresh Grindelia Floral Tops; see pages HYPE 1–5

★*Use only with physician's care.*

BRONCHITIS
Fresh Grindelia Floral Tops, Lungwort Extract, Fresh Pleurisy Root, Compounded Echinacea/ Goldenseal

COLDS
Compounded Echinacea/Goldenseal

COUGHS
In all cases use Compounded Wild Cherry with the following specifics:

Dry/Hacking
Yerba Santa, Fresh Sundew Extract, Slippery Elm, Lungwort Extract

Spasmodic
Fresh Sundew Extract, Fresh Lobelia Herb and Seed, Slippery Elm, Marshmallow Extract, Lungwort Extract

Irritative
Yerba Santa Leaf, Fresh Grindelia Floral Buds, Lungwort Extract

Whooping Cough
Fresh Sundew Extract, Fresh Lobelia Herb and Seed, Fresh Red Clover Blossoms

Congestive/Catarrhal
Fresh Eyebright Herb, Fresh Mullein Leaf, Fresh Bloodroot

Croup
Fresh Lobelia Herb and Seed, Fresh Sundew Extract

Emphysema
Cactus Grandiflorus Extract, Compounded Bugleweed/Motherwort, Fresh Lobelia Herb and Seed, Fresh Sundew Extract

Pleurisy
Fresh Pleurisy Root, Fresh Black Cohosh

Root, Fresh Stillingia Root, Fresh Lobelia Herb and Seed

Pneumonia
Compounded Echinacea/Goldenseal, Fresh Osha Root, Yerba Santa Leaf, Pleurisy Root, Compounded Lomatium

SKIN AND EPIDERMAL TISSUE
Herbal Agents Influencing the Functions of the Skin

ACNE

Oily
Compounded Red Clover, Fresh Yellow Dock Root, Compounded Juniper Berry, Compounded Milk Thistle/Yellow Dock

With Hormonal Origin
Compounded Red Clover, Sarsaparilla Root

Cystic
Compounded Red Clover, Fresh Burdock Root, Milk Thistle Seed, Compounded Juniper Berry, Compounded Echinacea/Red Root, Compounded Milk Thistle/Yellow Dock, Compounded Scudder's Alterative

BOILS/CARBUNCLES
Fresh Burdock Root, Compounded Red Clover, Compounded Echinacea/Red Root, Compounded Milk Thistle/Yellow Dock, Compounded Scudder's Alterative

BRUISES
St. John's Wort Flower Oil topically, Compounded Comfrey salve, Calendula Flower Oil, Compounded Comfrey Oil

BURNS
St. John's Wort Flower Oil topically, Compounded Comfrey Salve, Calendula Flower Oil

CANCER
Compounded Echinacea/Red Root, Fresh Black

Walnut Leaf and Hulls, Chaparral Leaf, Fresh
Plantain Leaf, Compounded Hoxsey/Red Clover,
Compounded Plantain/Goldenseal Salve topically

DERMATITIS
Contact
Compounded Comfrey Salve topically

ECZEMA
Compounded Red clover, Compounded Juniper
Berry, Fresh Burdock Root, Fresh Oregon Grape
Root, Compounded Echinacea, Fresh Thuja Leaf,
Compounded Milk Thistle/Yellow Dock

HERPES ZOSTER
Compounded Bloodroot/Celandine, Compounded
Lomatium, Compounded Skullcap/St. John's Wort,
Licorice Root Phytogel, St. John's Wort Extract

MELANOMAS
Compounded Echinacea/Red Root, Com-
pounded Plantain/Goldenseal Salve topically,
Fresh Turmeric Root, Fresh Thuja leaf

SHINGLES
Compounded Skullcap/St. John's Wort, Com-
pounded Lomatium, Compounded Bloodroot/
Celandine, Fresh Blue Flag Root

SORES
Fresh Thuja Leaf, Fresh Comfrey Root, Fresh
Marshmallow Root, Compounded Echinacea,
Compounded Comfrey Salve

PSORIASIS
Compounded Red Clover, Compounded Juniper
Berry, Fresh Burdock Root, Fresh Oregon Grape
Root, Fresh Blue Flag Root, Milk Thistle Seed,
Compounded Milk Thistle/Yellow Dock

WARTS
Fresh Thuja Leaf Oil topically

WOUNDS
Fresh St. John's Wort Oil topically, Compounded Comfrey Salve topically

URINARY SYSTEM
Herbal Agents Influencing the Renal Functions

BLADDER INFECTION
Compounded Usnea/Uva Ursi, Uva Ursi Solid Extract, Buchu Extract

CALCULI
Fresh Gravel Root, Bladderwrack Extract, Fresh Marshmallow Root, Compounded Juniper Berry, Madder Root

CYSTITIS
Fresh Marshmallow Root, Fresh Pipsissewa Herb, Fresh Horsetail Herb, Fresh Corn Silk, Fresh Gravel Root, Compounded Usnea/Uva Ursi, Buchu Extract

DROPSY
Fresh Horsetail Herb, Fresh Wild Carrot, Compounded Juniper Berry, Parsley Tea

ENURESIS
Fresh Plantain Leaf, Fresh Thuja Leaf, Fresh St. John's Wort Flower Buds, Fresh Corn Silk,

GRAVEL
Fresh Marshmallow Root, Fresh Pipsissewa Herb, Compounded Juniper Berry, Bladderwrack Extract, Fresh Gravel Root, Madder Root

INCONTINENCE
Fresh Thuja Leaf, Compounded Juniper Berry, Fresh St. John's Wort Flower Buds, Fresh Corn Silk, Fresh Plantain Leaf, Compounded Plantain/Buchu

KIDNEY INFECTION
Compounded Usnea/Uva Ursi, Uva Ursi Solid
Extract, Buchu Extract

KIDNEY STONES
Madder Root, Fresh Gravel Root, Fresh Marshmallow Root

NEPHRITIS
Fresh Goldenrod Flower Tops and Leaf, Fresh
Pipsissewa, Fresh Horsetail herb, Compounded
Juniper Berry

PROSTATITIS
Compounded Saw Palmetto, Fresh Thuja Leaf,
Fresh Cleavers Herb, Compounded Echinacea

SUPPRESSION
Compounded Juniper Berry, Fresh Goldenrod
Flowers and Herb, Fresh Cleavers Herb

Oone of the great principles of health and healing existing within the system of nature cure is proper elimination. Our physiology is designed with several major eliminative channels—the colon, the kidneys, the lungs, the skin, and the lymphatic system. Invariably, what influences the well-being of each of these systems is the capacity for one's metabolic processes to be carried out correctly. What follows is a brief summary of the herbal blends which when used together for a period of time work synergistically to restore balance to the metabolism and digestion and correct eliminative errors.

COMPOUNDED PSYLLIUM HUSK

Contents:

Psyllium Husks, Ayurvedic Triphala Powder, Marshmallow Root Powder, Licorice Root Powder, Ginger Root Powder.

Actions & Indications:

This formulation of herbs works remarkably well to revitalize digestion and improve absorption of food nutrients, while at the same time enhancing the elimination of wastes from the intestinal tract. The herbs in this blend promote a soothing bulk influence to the intestines. Triphala powder, an ancient Ayurvedic herbal blend, helps to enhance the functions of the organs of digestion and assimilation while revitalizing the entire metabolic processes. The effect of this synergistic blend of herbs is to remove putrefactive gases and wastes from the intestinal flora, expel mucous and endogenous toxins from the intestines, and relieve digestive and intestinal distress and irritation. Regular use of the Compounded Psyllium Husk each season promotes digestive and eliminative well-being.

Dosage: Use 1 teaspoon in 8–10 ounces of warm water and take 2 times daily. Shake well before using.

 COMPOUNDED ELIXIR OF BITTERS

Contents: Amalaki (Indian gooseberry), Turmeric Root, Milk Thistle Seed, Calamus Root, Wild Yam Root, Gentian Root, Fennel Seed, Cardamon Seed, Anise Seed, Bitter Orange Oil, Ginger Root, Extract of Sea Vegetation and Marine Algae.

Actions & Indications: Sluggish elimination is often a result of reduced secretions from the digestive organs and small intestine. Excessive refined foods generate stress upon the liver and pancreas and impede the natural metabolic functions. This is one reason why traditionally in almost every culture, herbal bitters are used. Compounded Elixir of Bitters represents a most effective blend of rejuvenative and carminative herbs which mildly stimulate and gently tonify the glands and digestive organs. Primary herbs in this formula are Turmeric Root and Indian Gooseberry. Both are indigenous to India, where they have been used traditionally to strengthen and protect the liver from endogenous toxins. Indian Gooseberry has also been shown to contain enzyme catalysts which improve nutrient absorption from the intestines. The other herbs in the formula work synergistically with these primary herbs to protect the liver from toxic overload, tonify the liver, gall bladder, and pancreas, and normalize stomach secretions. The volatile oils found in Fennel Seed, Cardamon Seed, and Anise Seed dispel gases from the stomach and intestines while Turmeric Root and Ginger Root normalize peristalsis and intestinal flora in the stomach and intestines.

Dosage: 1/2 teaspoon in warm water 3 times daily before meals.

COMPOUNDED JUNIPER BERRY

Contents: Fresh Juniper Berry, Fresh Spring Horsetail Herb, Fresh Corn Silk, Fresh Goldenrod Flowers and Leaf, Fresh Cleavers Herb, Fresh Marshmallow Root.

Actions & Indications: Our kidneys consume much energy in their efforts to remove metabolic wastes from the circulation. Periodic herbal renal support reduces the stress which accumulates throughout the renal system. In this formula, there are several cleansing herbs which have as their primary functions to gently stimulate renal excretions. In this cause, toxins circulating throughout the blood and lymph are carried out of the system. Toxins such as calculi, which build in the joints and tissues and which can cause edema and cystitis, impurities in circulation arising from digestive errors, and sediments and gravel which settle in the urinary system causing lumbar pain, painful urination, incontinence, etc.—all these are gradually corrected with the use of this herbal blend. As an adjunct in the Internal Cleansing Program, Compounded Juniper Berry mildly stimulates the kidneys, enabling better renal excretion to take place.

Dosage: Use 30–40 drops 3 times daily in warm water between meals.

COMPOUNDED RED CLOVER

Contents: Fresh Red Clover Blossoms, Fresh Stinging Nettle Leaf, Fresh Cleavers Herb, Fresh Yellow Dock Root, Fresh Burdock Root, Fresh Yarrow Flowers, Fresh Plantain Leaf, Fresh Licorice Root, and Prickly Ash Bark.

Actions & Indications: The influence of these herbs gradually alters the composition and constitution of the blood and lymph. This is accomplished through the removal of metabolic wastes which build up in the circulatory fluids and through the gentle nourishing and remineralizing effect that these herbs have upon the blood. Also, wasted tissues and cells are sloughed off and directed to eliminative channels for removal from the body. At the same time, new healthy tissue growth is encouraged with this herbal blend. Excessive impurities in the circulatory fluids are oftentimes the cause of metabolic changes in the body tissue and skin which may eventually give rise to tissue damage and dermatitis conditions such as eczema and psoriasis. Compounded Red Clover cools excess heat in the blood and liver which is associated with these disturbances. Compounded Red Clover is also effective for toxemia, lymph stagnation, lymph edema, swollen lymph glands, etc. Compounded Red Clover and Compounded Juniper Berry work synergistically together to correct blood impurities and remove them through proper eliminative channels.

Dosage: Use 30–40 drops 3–4 times daily in warm water between meals.

It is suggested that these four herbal compounds within this Internal Cleansing Program be used together for 6–8 weeks at the start of each season. During this time it is also suggested that the food intake be lighter, consisting of a higher percentage of whole grains and vegetables. Liquid intake (distilled water and fresh vegetable juice) should be increased. Daily stretching, brisk daily walking, and deep breathing exercises should accompany this program. Also, it would be very beneficial to take some warm water regularly (every 20 minutes) during the day while embarking upon this program.

The results should be noticeable: greater clarity, increased energy, improved digestion and elimination, and a greater sense of well being.

Aconite

Aconitum napellus
A valuable remedy for facial and trigeminal neuralgia. Also eases the arthritic or gouty pain often associated with neuralgia.
CAUTION: *For professional use only.*

Alfalfa Leaf

Medicago sativa
Alfalfa leaves are rich in protein, calcium and trace minerals, carotene, vitamins E and K. They are a rich source of weak plant phytoestrogens, useful in balancing the hormones when treating hyper- and hypo-estrongenism.

Angelica Root

Angelica archangelica
Angelica is a useful expectorant for coughs, bronchitis and pleurisy, especially when accompanied by colds, fever or flu. It also eases intestinal colic and flatulence, stimulates appetite and may be used in anorexia nervosa. It is helpful in easing rheumatic inflammations and acts as a urinary antiseptic in cystitis.

Arnica Flowers

Arnica latifolia
Taken internally, arnica is potentially toxic and can cause blistering of the intestinal mucosa. Externally, it is useful in treating any kind of pain or inflammation of the skin, as long as the skin is not broken. Use on bruises and sprains, and to relieve the pain and inflammation of phlebitis and rheumatism.

Ashwaganda

Withenia somnifera
This herb is considered the Ginseng of India in Ayurvedic medicine. It is adaptogenic and strengthens the body's power of resistance. It builds immunity and is useful as a general tonic to enhance virility and vitality.

Astragalus Root/ Huang Qi

Astragalus membranicus
Tones the spleen, useful in spleen deficiency

problems such as poor appetite, fatigue and diarrhea. Also useful for prolapse syndromes such as prolapsed uterus, stomach or anus, and also for uterine bleeding. Is an effective diuretic and promotes the discharge of pus.

Barberry Root Bark | *Berberis vulgaris*
An excellent remedy for correcting liver function and promoting bile flow. Use for gallbladder inflammation, gall stones and jaundice (when due to a congested liver). Barberry can reduce an enlarged spleen and can strengthen and cleanse a debilitated system.

Bayberry Bark | *Myrica cerifera*
Bayberry's astringent qualities make it valuable in treating diarrhea and dysentery. Useful for mucous colitis, as a gargle for sore throats and a douche for treating leukorrhea.

Black Cohosh Root | *Cimicifuga racemosa*
Black Cohosh is a powerful relaxant which is very useful in the treatment of rheumatic pains, osteo-arthritis, muscular and neurological pain and rheumatoid neuralgia. It also exerts a strong influence on the female reproductive system, normalizing menstruation and relieving menstrual cramps.

Black Haw Root & Tree Bark | *Viburnum prunifolium*
Black Haw Root is a powerful anti-spasmodic and nervine, acting particularly well on the uterus. It is used for dysmenorrhea, false labor pains and in threatened miscarriage. It can also relax peripheral blood vessels, and is used to reduce high blood pressure.

Black Walnut Hulls | *Juglans nigra*
A powerful remedy for expelling worms and also an antifungal, useful in treating candida, pinworms, ringworm and tapeworms. Also a mild laxative, and useful for treatment of skin problems such as eczema and herpes.

Bladderwrack Fronds | *Fucus vesiculosis*
Bladderwrack regulates thyroid function and is effective in treating underactive thyroid glands, goiter and all associated symptoms. Also helps relieve rheumatism and rheumatoid arthritis.

Blessed Thistle Herb | *Cnicus benedictus*
Primarily effective in treating female problems such as painful menstruation and associated headache. Stimulates menstruation, and is an excellent promoter of abundant breast milk especially when combined with Red Raspberry Leaves. Also stimulates gastric secretions, helping digestion.

Bloodroot | *Sanguinaria canadensis*
Bloodroot is valuable in treating congestive lung conditions such as chronic bronchitis and emphysema, acting to stimulate deficient peripheral circulation. At the same time it relaxes bronchial muscles and is useful in treating asthma, croup and laryngitis.

Blue Cohosh | *Caulophylum thalictroides*
An anti-spasmodic, Blue Cohosh is an excellent, safe herb for toning the uterus, easing false labor pains and dysmenorrhea, and can be used for threatened miscarriage. Its anti-spasmodic properties are also useful in treating colic, asthma or nervous coughs.

Blue Flag Root | *Iris versicolor*
Useful in treating a variety of skin diseases such as eczema and psoriasis, Blue Flag helps the skin by aiding the liver in its detoxifying work. Also valuable for constipation when it is caused by liver problems or biliousness.

Blue Vervain | *Verbena hastata*
Vervain is a tonic for the nervous system and is, at the same time, a sedative useful in easing tension, depression, hysteria and seizure. It promotes moderate perspiration useful in fevers and reduces

inflammation of the gall-bladder and is helpful in treating jaundice.

Boneset Herb | *Eupatorium perfoliatum*

Boneset is excellent in relieving the aches and pains from the flu. It is also helpful to the body in coping with any accompanying fever and clears mucous congestion from the upper respiratory tract.

Buchu Leaves | *Barosma betulina*

Acts as a diuretic and urinary antiseptic, helpful in any genito-urinary system infection such as cystitis, urethritis and prostatitis. Heals and soothes also.

Buckthorn Bark | *Rhamnus cathartica*

A stimulant and cathartic causing bowel movements, used mostly as a laxative but also as a bitter tonic to ease digestive problems.

Bugleweed Herb | *Lycopus virginica*

Used in treating over-active thyroid glands, especially when accompanied by tightness of breath, palpitations and shaking. An effective nervine, Bugleweed helps calm both palpitations and coughs that are of nervous origin.

Burdock Root | *Arctium lappa*

Burdock is quite effective in treating dry and scaly skin disorders such as psoriasis, dandruff and eczema, particularly when they are caused by a general systemic imbalance. It stimulates the digestive juices and bile secretion and therefore is useful in treating anorexia nervosa and digestion and appetite problems. Burdock also aids liver function and is used to heal cystitis.

Butterbur Root | *Petasites frigida*

Butterbur has spasmolytic and pain-relieving properties, with a beneficial effect on acute and chronic gastritis and gastroduodenitis, gastro-cardiac syndrome and painful spasms in the biliary tract.

Calamus Root | *Acorus calamus*

A powerful herb with a tonic effect on the stomach, promoting secretory activity and stimulating appetite. Very effective in treating appetite loss in conditions such as anorexia, childhood umbilical colic and all kinds of appetite disorders.

Calendula Flowers | *Calendula officinalis*

Calendula is one of the most valuable herbs in the treatment of external skin problems like slow-healing wounds, skins ulcers, inflammation or minor burns. Internally it reduces digestive inflammation and therefore is helpful in treating gastric and duodenal ulcers. Also useful for relieving indigestion and gall-bladder problems, and can help normalize delayed or painful menstruation.

California Poppy | *Escholzia californica*

Useful in treating sleeplessness and over-excitability in children, acting as a sedative. California Poppy is a non-addictive alternative to the Opium Poppy and may be used as a general anti-spasmodic.

Cascara Sagrada Bark | *Rhamnus purshiana*

Used as a laxative in treating chronic constipation, where it promotes peristalsis and tones relaxed digestive system muscles.

Catnip Herb | *Nepata cataria*

Commonly used in relieving colds and flu, Catnip promotes moderate perspiration and therefore is helpful in treating fevers and in particular acute bronchitis. Catnip is also anti-spasmodic and relieves stomach upset, dyspepsia, flatulence and colic. It is an excellent remedy for diarrhea in children, and is a useful sedative.

Celandine Tops & Roots | *Chelidonium majus*

Celandine promotes the flow of bile, stimulates the pancreas and is effective in gall-bladder problems, hepatitis, jaundice, gallstones and inflammatory conditions of the biliary system.

Chamomile Flowers, German | *Matricaria chamomilla*

Chamomile is an excellent nervine which relaxes and tones the nervous system and is especially useful in treating digestive problems such as gas, colic or ulcers produced by anxiety. It is safe for children of all ages in treating nervousness or teething pain, and can be added to the bath water. Chamomile is a sleep aid, a mild anti-microbial and an anti-catarrhal helpful in removing excess mucous in the sinus area.

Chaparral Leaf | *Larrea tridentata*

Chaparral sedates inflammation of the respiratory and intestinal tracts and relieves the pain of neuritis, sciatica and inflammations, and has antibacterial properties.

Chaste Tree Berry | *Vitex agnus-castus*

Normalizes and stimulates pituitary gland functions, particularly those of the female sex hormones; effective on dysmenorrhea, premenstrual stress and especially menopausal changes.

Chickweed Herb | *Stellaria media*

Useful in treating cuts, wounds, itching and irritation, particularly when the irritation is caused by eczema or psoriasis. Internally helpful with rheumatism.

Cinnamon Bark | *Cinnamonum zeylanicum*

This bark is a useful carminative agent aiding in the removal of gas in the digestive tract. It acts as a stomactic aiding the digestive processes. It is an effective styptic, and can be used as such with uterine hemorrhaging.

Cleavers Herb | *Galium aparine*

An excellent lymphatic system tonic with alliterative and diuretic properties, Cleavers works safely on a variety of lymphatic problems such as swollen glands (especially in tonsillitis and adenoid ailments). Useful in treating ulcers and tumors, since it aids lymphatic drainage and therefore detoxifies the tissue. Cleavers also is effective on painful urinary conditions such as cystitis.

Codonopsis Root/
Tang Shen Root

Codonopsis tangshen
Benefits the lungs and is helpful in treating chronic cough and shortness of breath. Also tones the spleen and helps deficient conditions such as tired limbs, diarrhea, vomiting and lack of appetite.

Cola Nut

Cola nitida
Stimulates the central nervous system and is helpful in cases of nervous debility, depression, and nervous diarrhea. May be used with other herbs to treat anorexia.

Collinsonia Root

Collinsonia canadensis
Collinsonia stimulates, cleanses and tones the mucous membranes of the digestive system and is helpful in gastro-enteritis with diarrhea and in hemorrhoids. It is also slightly astringent, relieving inflammations of the throat, flu, chronic pleurisy and colds.

Comfrey Leaf

Symphytum officinalis
An excellent demulcent which stimulates cell proliferation, useful in speeding the healing of gastric and duodenal ulcers, hiatus hernia and ulcerative colitis. Very high nutritive properties.

Comfrey Root

Symphytum officinalis
Same as Comfrey Leaf, but higher in mucilage which soothes and protects irritated or inflamed internal tissue.

Corn Silk

Zea mays
Corn Silk is a gentle diuretic, useful in treating urinary problems in children. It acts as a urinary demulcent when combined with others herbs to treat urinary ailments like cystitis, urethritis and prostatitis.

Cramp Bark

Viburnum opulus
An excellent anti-spasmodic, Cramp Bark works to relax muscular cramps in general and works on

the uterine and ovarian muscles in particular. By relaxing uterine muscles it relieves menstrual cramps and can help in threatened miscarriage. Its astringent properties are effective in treating excessive blood loss during menstruation and menopausal bleeding.

Damiana Herb | *Turnera diffusa*
Acts as a tonic on the central nervous system and the hormonal system. Used in treating depression and anxiety, particularly when influenced by sexual factors. Strengthens the male sexual system.

Dandelion Root | *Taraxacum officinalis*
Dandelion is an excellent, safe diuretic and liver tonic. Dandelion is a valuable diuretic because it is rich in potassium, a vital mineral often lost when the kidneys are stimulated by drugs. It is useful in treating water retention due to heart problems, inflammation and congestion of the liver and gall-bladder, and congestive jaundice.

Devil's Claw Root | *Harpagophytum procumbens*
Devil's Claw has anti-inflammatory properties which may help some cases of arthritis with inflammation and pain. Also acts as a hepatic in treating liver and gall bladder problems.

Devil's Club Root Bark | *Oplopanax horridum*
This herb is used as a blood sugar stabilizing agent. It is used routinely in the treatment of diabetes as a natural alternative to insulin.

Dong Quai Root/ Dang Gui | *Angelica sinensis*
Tones the blood and invigorates the circulatory system, acting on conditions such as palpitations, carbuncles or pain from congealed blood, abdominal pain and traumatic injuries. Also helps with irregular menstruation, amenorrhea and dysmenorrhea.

Dusty Miller | *Cineraria maritima*
Use in treating eye ailments such as conjunctivitis where it induces a low degree of hyperemia. Also helpful in the early stages of

senile cataract, especially when the vision is generally weak.

Elder Flowers

Sambucus canadensis

Colds and flu respond well to Elder Flowers, which are also helpful in treating upper respiratory tract inflammations such as sinusitis and hay fever.

Elecampane Root

Inula helenium

Useful in treating irritating bronchial coughs such as those that occur in bronchitis or emphysema, especially in children. Elecampane aids expectoration and at the same time has a soothing action. It can also be used in treating asthma, bronchitic asthma and tuberculosis.

Ephedra Twigs/ Ma Huang

Ephedra Sinica

Opens the pores and promotes perspiration, useful in treating chills, fever, headache and tight, floating pulse. Also helpful in controlling wheezing and relaxes the lungs. Promotes urination and reduces edema.

Eyebright Herb

Euphrasia officinalis

Eyebright has an anti-inflammatory action combined with astringent properties which make it a powerful treatment for congestive illnesses such as nasal catarrh and sinusitis. It is also used in treating eye conditions such as chronic or acute inflammations, stinging and weeping eyes and over-sensitivity to light.

Fennel Seed

Foeniculum vulgare

Excellent in treating stomach and intestinal problems such as flatulence, colic and lack of appetite. Calms bronchitis and coughs, and stimulates milk flow in nursing mothers.

Fennugreek Seed

Trigonella foenum-graecum

Valuable in healing and reducing inflammations in wounds; eases bronchitis and sore throats; soothes digestive problems and stimulates milk production in nursing mothers.

Feverfew Herb | *Chrysanthemum parthenium*
A valuable herb in the treatment of migraine headaches as well as relieving some of the accompanying symptoms such as nausea, depression and arthritic pain due to inflammation. Feverfew may also help ease dizziness, tinnitus, arthritis in its active inflammatory stage, and painful or sluggish menstruation.
CAUTION: *Do not use during pregnancy because of the stimulating action on the womb.*

Figwort | *Scrophularia nodosa*
Used primarily to treat skin problems such as psoriasis and eczema, acting as a general cleanser of the total body system. Acts as a mild laxative and diuretic. Avoid Figwort in cases of abnormally rapid heartbeat (tachycardia).

Fo-Ti Root/He Shou Wu | *Polygonum multiflorum*
Fo-Ti is astringent and helps treat conditions such as nocturnal emission, spermatorrhea or leukorrhea. It also tones the liver and kidneys as well as the blood.

Fringe Tree | *Chionanthus virginicus*
Valuable in treating all liver problems. Gall-bladder inflammation, gall-stones and jaundice all respond well to Fringe Tree's action of stimulating the flow of bile from the liver.

Garlic | *Allium sativum*
Garlic is one of the most effective anti-microbial herbs, with both anti-bacterial and anti-viral properties. It acts on respiratory infections such as chronic bronchitis, respiratory catarrh, recurrent colds and flu and is a powerful preventative for these conditions and for digestive infections as well. Garlic also lowers blood pressure, blood cholesterol levels and acts as a tonic on the cardiovascular system.

Gelsemium Root | *Gelsemium sempervirens*
Gelsemium is a cardiac sedative for extra systoles

and functional heart disease.
CAUTION: *For professional use only.*

Gentian Root | *Gentiana lutea*
Excellent in treating sluggish digestion and lack of appetite, as indicated by conditions like dyspepsia and flatulence. Gentian stimulates the appetite and digestion and promotes the production of saliva, gastric juices and bile.

Geranium Root | *Geranium maculatum*
Used primarily as an astringent in diarrhea, dysentery and hemorrhoids. May be used with other herbs to treat bleeding duodenal or gastric ulcers. Also acts to reduce blood loss during menstruation or uterine hemorrhage.

Ginger Root | *Zingiber officinalis*
Ginger acts as a peripheral circulation stimulant and is helpful in treating bad circulation, chilblains and cramps. It is also used as a remedy for digestive problems, sore throats and as a promoter of perspiration in treating fever.

Ginkgo Leaf | *Ginkgo biloba*
Ginkgo has a powerful effect on brain function and cerebral circulation and acts on wide range of vascular conditions. Some of these include vertigo, tinnitus, neurological disorders, Alzheimer's disease, memory and concentration problems, diminished intellectual capacity due to insufficient circulation, and complications of stroke and skull injuries.

Ginseng Root, Wild American and Woods-Grown American | *Panax quinquifolium*
Ginseng increases vitality and improves the body's resistance to a wide variety of illnesses and damaging external influences. Especially helpful to weak or elderly people.

Ginseng Root, Siberian | *Eleutherococcus senticosus*
Increases resistance to damaging external environmental factors and to illnesses, and increases vitality. Reduces incidence of flu, acute respiratory

disease, hypertension, ischemic heart disease, etc. Excellent as a general tonic.

Goldenrod Flowering Tops | *Solidago canadensis/odora*

A valuable herb in treating upper respiratory ailments such as cough, flu and bronchitis due to its stimulating and slightly astringent action on the mucous membranes. Goldenrod is also a urinary anti-inflammatory helpful in treating conditions like cystitis and urethritis.

Goldenseal Root | *Hydrastis canadensis*

Effective in all digestive problems from peptic ulcers to colitis, due to its tonic effects on the body's mucous membranes. Goldenseal is a powerful anti-microbial, improving all catarrhal conditions, especially those of the sinuses.

Gotu Kola Leaf & Root | *Hydrocotyle asiatica*

Gotu Kola is a stimulant to the central nervous system and is used to improve memory and treat fatigue.

Gravel Root | *Eupatorium purpureum*

Used in treating kidney stones (gravel), and also helpful in urinary infections such as cystitis and urethritis.

Grindelia Floral Buds | *Grindelia robusta*

Acting as a relaxant on smooth muscles and heart muscles, Grindelia is useful in treating asthmatic and bronchial conditions, especially when accompanied by rapid heart beat and nervousness. Blood pressure may go down with Grindelia.

Helonias Root | *Chamoelirium luteum*

An excellent tonic and strengthener of the reproductive systems for both sexes, although used primarily for women. Normalizes functions, tones and balances. Useful in delayed or absent menstruation, in ovarian pain, to prevent miscarriage and to ease vomiting associated with pregnancy.

Hops Strobile | *Humulus lupulus*
Hops relaxes the central nervous system and is an excellent remedy for insomnia, tension and anxiety. CAUTION: *Should be avoided in cases with marked depression, which may be accentuated by this herb.*

Horehound Herb | *Marrubium vulgare*
Valuable as an expectorant, promoting mucous production which can ease upper respiratory ailments such as bronchitis, whooping cough and colds.

Horse Chestnut | *Aesculus hippocastanum*
The actions of horse chestnut are astringent and anti-inflammatory, influencing largely the vessels of the circulatory system. It is a useful remedy for vascular fullness associated with hemorrhoids, varicose veins, rectal engorgement, phlebitis, and leg ulcers.

Horseradish Root | *Cochlearla armoracia*
This herb contains volatile oils effecting the sinus cavity and mucous membranes. It acts as a stimulant increasing secretions of these membranes and therefore is useful in sinus congestion. It is also useful in the treatment of laryngitis.

Horsetail Herb | *Equisetum arvense*
Horsetail acts on the genito-urinary system as an astringent which can reduce hemorrhaging and heal wounds. It is also a mild diuretic with toning and astringent properties, making it an effective treatment for incontinence and bed-wetting in children.

Hydrangea Root | *Hydrangea spp.*
Excellent in treating inflamed or enlarged prostate glands. Also acts as a sedative in urinary irritations and painful kidney stones associated with urinary infections.

Hyssop Flowering Herb | *Hyssopus officinalis*
Hyssop is useful in coughs, bronchitis and chronic catarrh due to its anti-spasmodic action. It also acts as nervine helpful in treating anxiety, hysteria and petit mal.

Jamaican Dogwood | *Piscidia erythrina*
A powerful sedative used primarily for insomnia due to nervous tension or pain. Helpful in treating the pain of neuralgia and migraine. Also relieves ovarian and uterine pain.

Jambul Seed | *Syzygium jambolana*
Jambul Seed is useful in treating diabetes, and also is used as a carminative, stomachic and diuretic.

Juniper Berry | *Juniperus communis*
An excellent diuretic with anti-microbial properties, useful in conditions such as cystitis. Its bitter action helps digestion and eases flatulent colic. CAUTION: *Avoid in any kidney disease and during pregnancy.*

Kava Kava Root | *Piper methysticum*
Kava Kava Root is a central nervous system depressant and a relaxant of the skeletal muscle which has no narcotic properties. It also anesthetizes the gastric and bladder mucosa and is useful in treating conditions such as irritable bladder syndrome.

Kelp Fronds | *Nereocystis luetkeana*
A very rich source of micro-nutrition, minerals and trace minerals. Especially high in iodine and potassium, useful for underactive thyroid function and for alkalizing blood chemistry.

Lavender Flowering Herb | *Lavendula officinalis*
Effective in treating headaches, especially those due to stress. Lavender is a valuable anti-depressant which also strengthens the nervous system and helps cases of nervous debility and exhaustion.

Lemon Balm | *Melissa officinalis*
Lemon Balm is a nervine which eases digestive tract spasms and is useful in flatulent dyspepsia. It also has mild anti-depressive properties and helps in tension, depression, migraine and anxiety-induced palpitations and insomnia.

Licorice Root	*Glycyrrhiza glabra* Acts on the endocrine system and the liver as an anti-hepatotoxic effective in treating hepatitis and cirrhosis. Licorice is also an expectorant and anti-inflammatory, useful in cough and bronchitis.
Life Root	*Senecio aurus* A tonic acting especially well on the female reproductive organs, Life Root is a safe, strengthening herb that is especially useful in treating menopausal disturbances. It also helps with delayed or suppressed menstruation and leukorrhea.
Ligustrum Berry/ Nu Zhen Zi	*Ligustrum lucidum* Nourishes and tones the liver and kidney, acting on conditions such as dizziness, spots in front of the eyes, lower back pain and tinnitus.
Lily of the Valley	*Convallaria magalis* Lily of the Valley is a cardiac tonic which increases coronary circulation and myocardial action, useful in treating conditions such as congestive heart failure, cardiac asthma and mitral insufficiency. Appropriate for all cardiac disturbances, especially conditions of incipient decompensation. CAUTION: *For professional use only.*
Linden Flowers	*Tilia spp.* Linden is valuable in the treatment of nervous tension and its relaxing properties are also helpful in some forms of migraine. Linden can prevent the development of arteriosclerosis and hypertension and is often used to treat high blood pressure when associated with arteriosclerosis and nervous tension.
Lobelia Herb & Seed	*Lobelia inflata* Lobelia is a valuable systemic relaxant, with a depressant action on the central and autonomic nervous systems. It is primarily used in bronchitic asthma and bronchitis, where it acts as a respiratory relaxant while at the same time stimulates catarrhal secretion and expectoration. CAUTION: *For professional use only.*

Lomatium Root

Lomatium dissectum

An effective anti-viral and anti-bacterial, especially useful in the treatment of respiratory and urinary infections. Lomatium stimulates the immune system and decreases inflammation.

Lungwort Lichen

Sticta pulmonaria

High in mucilage, and is indicated in respiratory conditions such as chronic bronchial cough and asthma. Also a bitter, promoting gastric juice secretions and useful for patients whose health is poor due to protracted cough.

Madagascar Periwinkle

Vinca rosea

A rich source of vincrisdine and vindblastine two alkaloids now being used as chemotherapeutic agents in the treatment of Hodgkin's disease.

Marshmallow Root

Althaea officinalis

Marshmallow soothes inflamed tissue in the digestive system, helping conditions such as inflammations of the mouth, gastritis, peptic ulceration and colitis.

Meadowsweet Herb

Filipendula ulmaria

An excellent remedy for digestive complaints such as nausea, heartburn, hyperacidity, gastritis and peptic ulcers. Also has gentle astringency useful for childhood diarrhea. Contains aspirin-like chemicals which relieve fever and rheumatic pain.

Melilot Flowering Herb

Melilotus officinalis

Melilot soothes the stomach and is useful for treating chronic flatulence, particularly following intestinal infections.

Milk Thistle Seed

Silybum marianum

Excellent as a liver tonic and in treating numerous liver and gall bladder conditions such as hepatitis and cirrhosis. May also reverse toxic liver damage and protect against hepatotoxic agents.

Mistletoe Herb	*Viscum flavenscens* Has gentle hypotensive properties affecting para-sympathetic stimulation and vasodilation, useful in treating symptoms associated with hypertension such as headaches, dizziness, loss of energy and irritability and in treating mild cases of hypertension. CAUTION: *For professional use only.*
Motherwort Flowering Herb	*Leonorus cardiaca* Motherwort is a nervine particularly effective in treating menstrual and uterine conditions, especially those influenced by anxiety or tension such as delayed or suppressed menstruation, menopausal changes and false labor pains. It is also effective in treating heart palpitations, especially caused by tension, and is an excellent heart tonic.
Mugwort Herb	*Artemesia vulgaris* Mugwort is a digestive aid, acting through the bitter stimulation of digestive juices. Mildly relaxing, it is useful in treating depression and nervous tension.
Mullein Leaf & Flowers	*Verbascum thapsus* Mullein is excellent in treating upper respiratory conditions such as bronchitis due to its tonic action on mucous membranes of the respiratory system. It also reduces inflammation of the trachea and at the same time soothes inflamed tissues.
Myrrh Gum	*Commiphora molmol* Myrrh's anti-microbial action is especially effective in mouth infections such as gingivitis and phyorrhea, in sinusitis, laryngitis and respiratory complaints. Often used in treating the common cold. Also helpful in systemic conditions like boils, glandular fever and brucellosis.
Nettle Leaf	*Urtica dioica* Nettles affect a wide range of ailments and act as a tonic and general detoxifying remedy for the whole body. They excel in treating some cases of rheumatism and arthritis, and also are beneficial in

all varieties of eczema, particularly childhood
eczema and in cases caused by nervous tension.

Night-Blooming
Cereus

Cactus grandiflorus
Night Blooming Cereus is a stimulating cardiac
tonic which raises the blood pressure and regulates
the pulse. Effective in conditions such cardiac
weakness, low blood pressure, anemia and angina.

Oats,
Wild Milky Seed

Avena sativa
An excellent remedy for strengthening the
entire nervous system, Oats are used in treating
nervous debility, exhaustion when associated with
depression, and stress

Osha Root

Ligusticum porteri
An excellent herb for treating viral infections,
producing thorough perspiration and elimination
of toxins. Useful for bronchial inflammations and
sore throats, acting to soothe sore tissues while also
promoting expectoration.

Oregon Grape Root

Berberis aquafolium
Acts as a tonic on the liver and gall-bladder and
can remedy chronic and scaly skin problems such
as psoriasis and eczema which are caused by systemic imbalances. Also helpful for stomach and
gall-bladder conditions, especially when associated
with vomiting and nausea.

Parsley Leaf & Root

Petroselinum crispum
Parsley is a diuretic, can ease flatulence and the
accompanying colic pains, and can stimulate the
menstrual process.
CAUTION: *Do not use in medicinal dosage during
pregnancy.*

Passionflower

Passiflora incarnata
As a sedative, Passionflower is the preferred
herb for treating insomnia and leaves no
hangover. As an anti-spasmodic, it is helpful in
Parkinson's Disease, asthma (with much
spasmodic activity), seizures and hysteria. It

relieves nerve pain in conditions like neuralgia and shingles.

Pau D'Arco Inner Bark | *Tabebuia impetiginosa*
A South American tree bark which has strong anti-fungal and anti-yeast properties, used as a blood alterative, prophylactically and in chronic health imbalances.

Pennyroyal | *Mentha pulegium*
Useful primarily as a uterine stimulant, to strengthen uterine contractions during labor and to start the menstrual process. Also eases flatulence and abdominal colic caused by wind.
CAUTION: *Avoid during pregnancy.*

Peppermint Leaf | *Mentha piperita*
Peppermint relaxes the muscles of the digestive system, relieving conditions like flatulence, intestinal colic and flatulent dyspepsia. It also acts as a mild anesthetic to the stomach wall and is useful in treating nausea and vomiting. It can relieve nasal catarrh and is used in colds, fevers and flu. Peppermint is also a nervine, helpful in easing painful periods and lessening anxiety.

Periwinkle Herb | *Vinca minor*
Excellent as an astringent, used primarily in treating excessive menstrual flow and similar problems in the urinary system such as hematuria. Its astringency reduces the loss of fluid or blood in digestive conditions such as colitis or diarrhea. It also is effective in treating nose bleeds, bleeding gums, mouth ulcers or sore throats.

Pipsissewa Herb | *Chimaphila umbellata*
A urinary antiseptic and a diuretic with a beneficial effect on the liver, kidney and bladder. Pipsissewa also has astringent properties making it useful in treating conditions such as diarrhea.

Plantain Leaf & Corm | *Plantago lanceolata*
Plantain is an astringent, acting to reduce fluids in

a variety of conditions including diarrhea, dysentery, hemorrhoids, excessive menstrual flow and hematuria. It is also a gentle expectorant which soothes inflamed membranes, helping in coughs, mild bronchitis and inflammation of the intestinal tract.

Pleurisy Root　*Asclepias tuberosa*
　　Valuable in treating all kinds of respiratory infections such as pneumonia, pleurisy, flu and bronchitis. Pleurisy Root reduces inflammation, promotes moderate perspiration and aids expectoration.

Poke Root　*Phytolacca americana*
　　Poke Root is a remedy for upper respiratory infections, useful in treating cough, tonsillitis, laryngitis, swollen glands and mumps. It cleans the lymphatic glands throughout the body and is especially helpful in mastitis. It is also used for rheumatism. CAUTION: *In large doses Poke Root is a powerful emetic and purgative (causes vomiting). For professional use only.*

Prickly Ash Bark　*Xanthoxylum clava-herculis*
　　Stimulates the circulation, lymphatic system and mucous membranes; effective in chilblains, leg cramp, varicose veins and ulcers, rheumatism and skin diseases.

Propolis/Bee-Harvested Tree Resin　A strong anti-microbial, anti-bacterial and anti-viral agent used topically and in the treatment of wounds, injuries and infections. Very useful as a first-aid remedy.

Pygeum Bark　*Pygeum africanum*
　　Effective in the treatment of benign prostate hyperplasia, or prostatic inflammation.

Red Clover Blossoms　*Trifolium pratense*
　　A safe and effective treatment for childhood eczema. Also useful for chronic skin problems in children and adults such as psoriasis. An expectorant and antispasmodic, Red Clover works especially well on whooping cough and also on coughs and bronchitis.

Red Raspberry Leaves	***Rubus idaeus*** Valuable as a strengthener and toner of the womb during pregnancy, and helpful in restraining hemorrhage during labour and assisting contractions. Its astringent action is also helpful in reducing fluids for a variety of other conditions including diarrhea, leukorrhea and mouth problems such as bleeding gums and inflammations.
Red Root	***Ceanothus americanus*** Red Root stimulates lymph and intertissue fluid circulation and is effective on tonsil inflammations, sore throats, enlarged lymph nodes and for shrinking non-fibrous cysts. It also has astringent properties useful in stopping menstrual hemorrhage, nosebleeds, bleeding piles, hemorrhoids and capillary ruptures from vomiting or coughing.
Rose Hips	***Rosa rugosa*** An astringent affecting primarily the kidneys, bladder and colon, controlling diarrhea and reducing urine excretion and intestinal leakage. Helps to stabilize the kidneys.
Rosemary Leaf	***Rosmarinus officinalis*** Rosemary calms and tones the digestive system, helping ease conditions like flatulent dyspepsia. It also helps with nervous tension which may manifest in headache or depression.
Rue	***Ruta graveolens*** Rue acts primarily on the uterus, bringing on suppressed menstruation; it is a powerful abortifacient. It is also used to relax the muscles of the digestive system, easing griping and bowel tension. The anti-spasmodic action also helps to stop spasmodic coughs. CAUTION: *Avoid during pregnancy.*
Sage Leaf	***Salvia officinalis*** Sage is excellent in reducing inflammations of the mouth, throat and tonsils and is used in treating

ailments such as gingivitis, mouth ulcers, laryngitis and tonsillitis. It is also helpful in dyspepsia.
CAUTION: *Avoid during pregnancy.*

Sarsaparilla Root | *Smilax officinalis v. omata*
Gradually restores the proper functioning of the body, correcting a wide range of systemic problems. These include scaling skin conditions such as psoriasis, and rheumatic conditions. Especially useful for rheumatoid arthritis.

Saw Palmetto Berry | *Serenoa repens*
Acts as a tonic and strengthener of the male reproductive system, and is helpful in treating enlarged prostate glands. Also useful in genitourinary tract infections.

Schizandra Berry/ Wu Wei Zi | *Schizandra chinensis*
Strengthens and quickens reflexes, stimulates respiration and is useful in promoting labor. Also reduces perspiration, stops coughing and diarrhea.

Sheep Sorrel | *Rumex acetosella*
This herb has been popularized as a key ingredient in Renée Caisse's Essiac formula. Eclectic references suggest it has a marked influence on "tissue of lower organization" and thus is useful for degenerative tissues throughout the body.

Shepherd's Purse | *Capsella Bursa-pastoris*
Acts as an astringent in conditions such as diarrhea, wounds, nose bleeds and excessive menstrual flow, while at the same time is useful in stimulating suppressed menstruation. Also useful as a gentle diuretic.

Skullcap Herb | *Scutellaria laterifolia*
An excellent nervine for a wide range of ailments. Skullcap relaxes while also revivifying the central nervous system. Valuable in treating seizure, hysteria and epilepsy. A safe treatment for easing pre-menstrual tension.

Chinese Skullcap | *Scutellaria baicalensis*
Chinese Skullcap is anti-microbial, antipyretic and anti-inflammatory. It is used for treating high fevers and accompanying irritability, thirst, cough and expectoration of sputum. Also acts on the digestive system, easing diarrhea or dysentery-like disorders, and helps with painful urinary dysfunction.

Skunk Cabbage Root | *Symplocarpus foetidus*
An effective anti-spasmodic for lung ailments, easing and relaxing cough or lung tension in conditions such as asthma, bronchitis and whooping cough. Also promotes moderate perspiration useful in treating fevers.

Slippery Elm Inner Bark | *Ulmus rubra*
Slippery Elm is useful in treating digestive conditions with inflamed mucous membrane linings such as gastritis, gastric or duodenal ulcer, enteritis and colitis, where it has a soothing, demulcent action.

Spearmint | *Mentha spicata*
This herb is used in a similar way as peppermint, only somewhat milder. It is an effective carminative aid to dispell gas in the digestive tract, and can be used as a mild diaphoretic.

Spilanthes Flowering Tops & Root | *Spilanthes acmella*
Promotes secretion of saliva and is useful in improving the appetite and digestive functions, overcoming nausea and vomiting and eases flatulence.

Squaw Vine | *Mitchella repens*
An excellent herb to take during pregnancy, to prepare the uterus and the whole body for a safe childbirth. Also used to relieve painful periods. Its astringency is effective in treating colitis, especially when accompanied by excess mucous.

St. John's Wort | *Hypericum perforatum*
A sedative and pain reducer useful in treating neuralgia, anxiety, depression and in particular,

irritability and tension due to menopausal changes. Also helpful in easing the pain of fibrositis, sciatica and rheumatic pain.

Stillingia Root

Stillingia sylvatica

An excellent alterative acting primarily on the lymphatic and secretory systems, useful in treating any kind of laryngeal irritation, bronchitis, and syphilis.

Tansy

Tanacetum vulgare

Acting primarily on the digestive system, tansy is effective in eliminating roundworm and threadworm but is dangerous to use over a long period of time. Eases dyspepsia and is an enema treatment for children. Also may be used to stimulate menstruation. CAUTION: *Avoid during pregnancy. For professional use only.*

Thuja Leaf

Thuja occidentalis

Acts as an expectorant, useful in treating bronchial catarrh. When the catarrh is accompanied by heart weakness, Thuja Leaf is helpful since it also is a systemic stimulant, but it should be avoided if the catarrh is due to over-stimulation. Also stimulates menstruation. CAUTION: *Avoid during pregnancy.*

Thyme Leaf

Thymus vulgaris

Stimulates and soothes the digestive system, helpful in easing dyspepsia and sluggish digestion. Its anti-microbial action is effective in sore throats, laryngitis, respiratory and digestive infections. An excellent cough remedy for bronchitis, whooping cough and asthma.

Turmeric Root

Curcuma longa

Turmeric Root is a powerful gall-bladder stimulant, promoting the flow of bile. Also stimulates gastric juices. A powerful anti-oxidant, anti-inflammatory and anti-hepatotoxic herb, useful in the treatment of inflammatory conditions such as diabetes, hepatitis, liver disorders and skin conditions.

Usnea Lichen | *Usnea spp.*
Old man's beard, as it is sometimes called, contains usneic acid, which is a strong respiratory and urinary antibiotic. This herb is useful in the treatment of bronchitis, pleurisy, and other respiratory infections, as well as being an effective treatment of urinary tract, kidney, and bladder infections.

Uva Ursi Leaf | *Arctostaphylos uva ursi*
Soothes, tones and strengthens the membranes of the urinary system and is helpful in gravel or ulceration of the kidney or bladder, pyelitis and cystitis.

Valerian Root | *Valeriana officinalis*
An excellent nervine for treating anxiety and tension, and a gentle, safe sleep aid. Valerian's antispasmodic action makes it a strong muscle relaxing used in muscle cramping, uterine cramps and intestinal colic.

Venus' Flytrap | *Dionaea muscipula*
Stimulates and modulates the immune system, and reduces the growth rate of tumor tissue while increasing the number and activity of T-helper cells and other factors of the immune system. Helpful in treating conditions such as cancer, HIV, AIDS or other degenerative or infectious diseases.

White Oak Bark | *Quercus alba*
A powerful astringent used primarily in treating diarrhea; also useful in dysentery and hemorrhoids although it may be too strong for some conditions.

Willow Bark | *Salix spp.*
A natural form of aspirin and used on similar conditions such as aches and pains, rheumatism, gout and fever.

Wild Cherry Bark | *Prunus serotina*
Wild Cherry is a strong sedative for the cough

reflex and is part of the treatment for bronchitis, whooping cough and all kinds of irritating cough. May also be combined with other herbs to treat asthma.

Wild Indigo Root	***Baptisia tinctoria***

Wild Indigo's anti-microbial action makes it useful in treating focused infections, particularly those of the ear, nose and throat. Also used systemically to treat enlarged and inflamed lymph glands.

Wild Yam Root	***Dioscorea villosa***

A valuable anti-spasmodic used to relieve intestinal colic, diverticulitis, dysmenorrhea and ovarian and uterine pains. Excellent as an anti-inflammatory in treating rheumatoid arthritis.

Witch Hazel Bark, Twigs & Leaf	***Hamamelis virginiana***

Witch Hazel is used as an astringent to ease bleeding, hemorrhoids, bruises, inflamed swellings, dysentery and varicose veins. It controls diarrhea.

Wood Betony	***Stachys betonica***

Wood Betony targets the nervous system and acts as a tonic and general relaxer. It is useful for anxiety and nervous tension associated with occasional headache and hypertension.

Wormseed	***Chenopodium ambrosiodes***

Wormseed is an aromatic herb with volatile oils effective in the treatment of worms, amoebas, and parasites. It is also a strong bitter agent influencing the secretions of the GI tract.

Wormwood Herb	***Artemisia absinthum***

Wormwood's bitter action stimulates the digestive system, helping indigestion, especially when caused by gastric juice problems. A strong herb for treating worm infestations, particularly roundworm and pinworm.

Yarrow Flowers	***Achillea millefolium***

Promotes moderate perspiration helpful in

relieving fevers. Lowers blood pressure, stimulates digestion and tones blood vessels. Useful in treating urinary infections such as cystitis.

Yellow Dock Root | *Rumex crispus*
A valuable herb for treating chronic skin conditions such as psoriasis. Promotes the flow of bile and is used for jaundice when caused by congestion, is a blood cleanser and a remedy for constipation.

Yerba Santa Leaf | *Eriodictyon californicum*
Yerba Santa is an expectorant and bronchial dilator, useful primarily in treating upper respiratory ailments such as asthma, pneumonia and coughs. Also effective for mild bladder and urethra infections.

Yohimbe Bark | *Corynanthe yohimbe*
A rich source of strong alkaloids which block the uptake of neuro-transmitters at Alpha-2 receptor sites, effective in dieting and weight management, Parkinson's disease, impotence and lack of libido.

Yucca Root | *Yucca spp.*
Yucca is an anti-inflammatory, useful in treating joint inflammation and arthritic pain. Can have a laxative effect.

NOTES

NOTES

NOTES

NOTICE

The following Naturopathic Desk Reference (NDR) section is an introduction to a much more elaborate *Protocol Journal of Botanical Medicines*. The NDR provides the reader with insights into useful and practical alternatives to common allopathic drugs. In the forthcoming quarterly *Protocol Journal*, available in April 1994, the information is expanded to include complete therapeutic protocols that present Western allopathic practices and naturopathic, Ayurvedic, and Chinese practices to the same rigorous standards as traditional medical journals. Drawing from ten databases of published research conducted around the world, the peer-reviewed *Protocol Journal* will present etiologies, treatments, toxicologies, pharmacologies, nutritional information, "nature cure" applications, journal references, and physician reviews. Annual subscriptions will cost $36.00.

If you would like to receive more information about the Protocol Journal of Botanical Medicines, please fill out and return the form that follows the NDR section. Thank you.

•
NATUROPATHIC
Desk Reference
•

GYNECOLOGICAL CONDITIONS

Physiology of Hormones
Premenstrual Syndrome
Menopause (estrogen
 replacement)
Amenorrhea
Dysmenorrhea
Menorrhagia
Ovarian Cysts
Uterine Fibroids
Endometriosis
Fibrocystic Breasts/Mastitis
Infertility

Pregnancy: *Herbal*
 Contraindications
 Threatened Miscarriage
 Anemia
 Nausea
 Constipation
 Hemorrhoids
 Urinary Tract Infections
 Hypertension
 Leg Cramps

BOTANICAL MATERIA MEDICA

Simple Herbs

Achellia millefolium
 (Yarrow)
Atetris farinosa (True
 Unicorn)
Althaea off. (Marshmellow)
Angelica sinesis (Dong
 Quai)
Arctium lappa (Burdock)
Avena sativa (Oats)
Berberis aquafolium
 (Oregon Grape)
Capsella bursa-pastoris
 (Shepherd's Purse)
Caulophyllum thalictroides
 (Blue Cohosh)
Chamaelirium luteum
 (False Unicorn/Helonias)
Cimicifuga racemosa (Black
 Cohosh)
Dioscorea villosa (Wild
 Yam)
Equisetum arvense
 (Horsetail)
Glycyrrhiza glabra
 (Licorice)
Hydrastis canadensis
 (Goldenseal)

Hyssopus off. (Hyssop)
Leonurus cardiaca
 (Motherwort)
Medicago sativa (Alfalfa)
Mentha piperita
 (Peppermint)
Mitchella repens (Squaw
 Vine)
Phytolacca americana
 (Poke)
Piscidia Erythrina (Jamaican
 Dogwood)
Pulsatilla
Rumex crispus (Yellow
 Dock)
Salvia off. (Sage)
Scutellaria lateriflora
 (Skullcap)
Senicio aureus (Life Root)
Smilax officinalis
 (Sarsaparilla)
Taraxacum officinalis
 (Dandelion)
Urtica diocia (Nettles)
Valeriana sitchensis
 (Valerian)

Simple Herbs (cont.)
Viburnum opulus (Cramp Bark)
Viburnum prunifolium (Black Haw)
Zingiber officinalis (Ginger)

Compounds
Compounded Vitamin C
   Elixir
Compounded Devils Club
Compunded Dong Quai
Compounded
   Echinacea/Red Root
Compounded
   Feverfew/Jamaican
   Dogwood
Compounded
   Fraxinus/Ceanothus

Compounded
   Gelsemium/Phytolacca
Compounded Passiflorus
   Elixir
Compounded Bitters Elixir
Compounded Usnea/Uva
   Ursi
Compounded Vitex Elixir
Compounded Vitex/Alfalfa

Supplements & Specialty Items
Alfalfa Solid Extract
Bromalian
Calcium
Carotenoids
Castor Oil
Evening Primrose Oil
Lactobacillus

Manganese
Magnesium
Poke Root Oil
Tyrosine
Vitamin B 6
Vitamin K
Flax Seed Oil

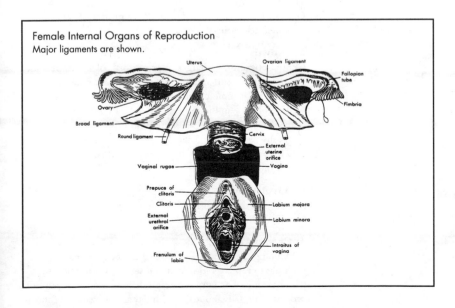

Female Internal Organs of Reproduction
Major ligaments are shown.

THE MENSTRUAL CYCLE

Menstrual Phase (menstruation): Days 1 to 4
- Estrogen and progesterone withdrawn before onset of menstrual flow.
- Shedding of endometrial lining.

Proliferative (follicular) phase: Days 5 to 14
- Regrowth of endometrial tissue.
- Secretion of follicle-stimulating hormone (FSH) by the pituitary gland.
- Development in ovary of a mature Graafian follicle containing a mature ovum.
- Secretion of increasing amounts of estrogen by Graafian follicle.
- Suppression of FSH when estrogen level becomes high, leading to secretion of luteinizing hormone (LH) by pituitary gland.

Secretory (luteal) phase: Days 15 to 25–28
- Rupture of Graafian follicle, releasing ovum (ovulation), starts the the secretory phase.
- Movement of ovum through fallopian tube to uterus.
- Formation of corpus luteum at site of ruptured Graafian follicle.
- Production of progesterone by corpus luteum.
- Stimulation by progesterone of endometrial cell growth.
- Significant decrease in progesterone level if implantation does not occur; menstrual phase then begins again.

OOGENESIS

There are two ovaries. These produce the female germ cells. The production of ova is a cyclical process called oogenesis.

1) Formation
Germinal epithelium: in development groups of cells migrate into stroma.

2) Growth
Central oogonium enlarges in primordial follicle to become primary oocyte surrounded by follicular cells which multiply to become cumulus oophorus (attaching ovum to wall of follicle) and membrana granulosa which together with cells of theca interna, secrete hormone estrogen— partly stored in liquor folliculi in enlarging cavity of developing Graafian follicle—partly absorbed into blood vessels of theca interna.

(3) Ovulation
About 14th day of normal 28–day menstrual cycle, a mature Graafian follicle ruptures to expel ovum.

4) Corpus Luteum
Remaining membrana granulosa and theca interna cells multiply to replace blood clot and secrete hormone progesterone. The corpus luteum shrinks and its output of progesterone falls about the 24th day if fertilization of the

shed ovum does not occur. For simplicity the development of only one Graafian follicle is shown here. Several grow in each cycle but in the human subject only one Follicle ruptures. The others atrophy, i.e., one mature ovum is shed each month.

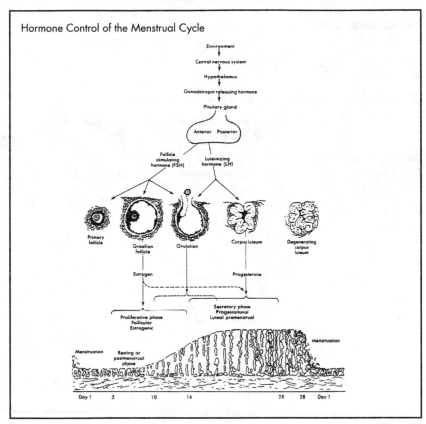

Hormone Control of the Menstrual Cycle

SIGNS & SYMPTOMS OF PREMENSTRUAL SYNDROME (PMS)

Behavioral

Nervousness, anxiety, and irritability

Mood swings and mild to severe personality changes

Fatigue, lethargy, and depression

Gastrointestinal

Abdominal bloating

Diarrhea and/or constipation

Change in appetite (craving of sugar)

Female

Tender and enlarged breasts

Uterine cramping

Altered libido

General
Headache
Backache
Acne
Edema of fingers and ankles

HORMONAL PATTERNS OF PREMENSTRUAL SYNDROME

- Plasma estrogens are elevated and plasma progesterone levels are reduced 5–10 days before menses

- Prolactin levels are elevated in most PMS women

- Follicle Stimulating Hormone (FSH) levels are elevated 6–9 days prior to the onset of the menses

- Aldosterone levels are marginally elevated 2–8 days prior to the onset of the menses.

BOTANICAL THERAPIES FOR PREMENSTRUAL SYNDROME

PMS–A (Anxiety):
Metabolize Estrogen / Stimulate Progesterone

Vites agnus castus (Chaste Tree Berry)	20–30 drops t.i.d.
Dioscorea villosa (Wild Yam)	30–40 drops t.i.d.
Chamoelirium luteum (Helonias Root)	20–30 drops t.i.d.
Evening Primrose Oil	500 mg q.i.d.
Vitamin B-6	100 mg b.i.d.
Compounded Elixir of Bitters	1 teaspoon after meals in small amount of water
Compounded Elixir of Passionflower	1 teaspoon t.i.d.
Compounded Vitamin C Elixir	1 teaspoon b.i.d.

PMS–C (Cravings):
Promote Digestion / Stimulate Progesterone / Decrease Inflammatory PGE

Evening Primrose Oil	500 mg q.i.d.
Compounded Bitters Elixir	1 teaspoon after meals in warm water
Compounded Devil's Club	20–30 drops t.i.d.
Angelica sinensis (Dong Quai Root)	30 drops t.i.d.
Taraxacum officinalis (Dandelion Root & Leaf)	30–40 drops t.i.d.
Bromalain	500 mg t.i.d.

PMS–D (Depression):
Increase Estrogen / Support Adrenals

Compounded Dong Quai	30–40 drops t.i.d.
Glycyrrhiza glabra (Licorice Root)	40 drops t.i.d.

Medicago sativa
(Alfalfa Solid Extract)   1/2 teaspoon t.i.d.
Compounded Elixir of Passionflower   1 teaspoon t.i.d.
Tyrosine   300 mg b.i.d.

PMS–H (Hyperhydration):
Balance Hormones/Support Adrenals

Compounded Dong Quai
                    30–40 drops t.i.d. during Follicular phase
Compounded Elixir of Vitex
                        1 teaspoon t.i.d. during luteal Phase
Compounded Elixir of Bitters
                        1 teaspoon after meals in warm water
Glycyrrhiza glabra
(Licorice Root)   40 drops t.i.d.
Dioscorea villosa
(Wild Yam)   30 drops t.i.d.
Lactobacillus

PREMENSTRUAL SYNDROME
SUB-GROUPS

SUB-GROUP	SYMPTOMS	MECHANICS	PREVALENCE
PMS–A (Anxiety)	Anxiety Irritability Mood Swings Nervous Tension	↑ Estrogen ↓ Progesterone	65–75%
PMS–C (Craving)	Appetite Headache Fatigue Dizziness	↑ Carb. Tolerance ↓ Progesterone ↑ PGEI	24–35%
PMS–D (Depression)	Depression Crying Confusion Forgetfulness	↓ Blood Estrogen ↑ Progesterone Elevated adrenal	23–37%
PMS–H (Hyperhydration)	Fluid Retention Weight Gain Breast Tenderness Bloating	Aldosterone	65–72%

BOTANICAL
THERAPIES FOR
GYNECOLOGICAL
CONDITIONS

AMENORRHEA
Absense of or delayed menses

Compounded Dong Quai	30 drops t.i.d.
Compounded Elixir of Vitex	1 teaspoon t.i.d.

Compound of the following herbs:

Caulophylum thalictroides (Blue Cohosh)	20 drops t.i.d.
Chamoelirium luteum (Helonias Root)	20 drops t.i.d.
Senecio aurus (Life Root)	20 drops t.i.d.
Leonurus cardiaca (Motherwort)	20 drops t.i.d.
Zingiber officinalis (Ginger Root)	5 drops t.i.d.
Dioscorea villosa (Wild Yam)	20 drops t.i.d.

DYSMENORRHEA
Painful Menstruation

Compounded Dong Quai

30 drops t.i.d. during Follicular phase

Compounded Elixir of Vitex

1 teaspoon t.i.d. during Luteal phase

Viburnum prunifolium (Black Haw)	30 drops t.i.d.
Caulophylum thalictroides (Blue Cohosh)	20 drops t.i.d.
Piscidia erythrina (Jamaican Dogwood)	30 drops t.i.d.
Scutellaria lateriflora (Skullcap)	30 drops t.i.d.

Note: Take the above 4 herbs during the onset of menstrual pain. If necessary, take the herbs more often.

Compounded Feverfew/Jamaican Dogwood

40 drops q.i.d.
or more frequently during menstrual pain.

MENORRHAGIA
Excessive or prolonged menstrual bleeding

Compounded Elixir of Vitex	1 teaspoon t.i.d.
Angelica sinensis (Dong Quai Root)	30 drops t.i.d.
Capsella bursa–pastoris (Shepherd's Purse)	40 drops q.i.d.
Achellia millefolium (Yarrow)	20 drops q.i.d.
Hydrastis canadensis (Goldenseal Root)	20 drops t.i.d.

OVARIAN CYSTS

Scudder's Alterative	30 drops t.i.d.
Compounded Echinacea/Red Root	30–40 drops t.i.d.
Compounded Fraxinus/Ceanothus	30–40 drops q.i.d.
Compounded Gelsemium/Phytolacca	15 drops q.i.d.

Compound the following four herbs:

Taraxacum officinalis (Dandelion Root)	20 drops q.i.d.
Glycyrrhiza glabra (Licorice Root)	20 drops t.i.d.
Rumex crispus (Yellow Dock Root)	20 drops t.i.d.
Arctium lappa (Burdock Root)	20 drops t.i.d.

Carotenoids	150,000–300,000 IU daily
Castor Oil Packs	over ovaries 3–5 times/week

If pain is present use:

Valeriana sitchensis (Valerian Root)	1 teaspoon q.i.d.
Viburnum opulus (Cramp Bark)	30 drops t.i.d.

UTERINE FIBROIDS

Scudder's Alterative	30 drops t.i.d.
Compounded Echinacea/Red Root	30–40 drops t.i.d.
Compounded Fraxinus/Ceanothus	30–40 drops q.i.d.
Compounded Gelsemium/Phytolacca	15 drops q.i.d.
Compounded Vitex Elixir	1 teaspoon t.i.d.
Dong Quai Root	30 drops t.i.d.
Carotenoids	150,000–300,000 IU daily

Compound:

Urtica dioica (Nettles)	50 drops t.i.d.
Arctium lappa (Burdock Seed)	20 drops t.i.d.
Taraxacum officinalis (Dandelion Root)	20 drops t.i.d.
Berberis aquafolium (Oregon Grape)	20 drops t.i.d.
Poke Root Oil	Rub into uterus before bed
Castor Oil packs	Apply over pelvis 3–5 times/week
Sitz baths	Daily

Herbal Suppositories:

White Oak Bark
Goldenseal Root
Tea Tree Oil

ENDOMETRIOSIS

Scudder's Alterative	30 drops t.i.d.
Compounded Fraxinus/Ceanothus	30–40 drops q.i.d.
Compounded Echinacea/Red Root	30–40 drops t.i.d.
Compounded Vitex Elixer	1 teaspoon t.i.d.
Dong Quai Root	30 drops t.i.d.
Compounded Gelsemium/Phytolacca	15 drops q.i.d.

For Pain:

Compounded Feverfew/Jamaican Dogwood	
	50–60 drops q.i.d. as needed for pain
Carotenoids	150,000–300,000 IU daily
Sitz Baths	Daily before bed
Castor Oil Packs over pelvis	3 times/week.
Evening Primprose Oil	500 mg q.i.d.

FIBROCYSTIC BREASTS/MASTITIS

Scudder's Alterative	30 drops t.i.d.
Compounded Echinacea/Red Root	30–40 drops q.i.d.
Phytolacca americana	
(Poke Root)	10 drops t.i.d.

Compound:

Arctium lappa (Burdock Seed)	20 drops t.i.d.
Taraxacum officinalis (Dandelion Root)	20 drops t.i.d.
Hydrastis canadensis (Goldenseal Root)	20 drops t.i.d.
Carotenoids	150,000–300,000 IU daily
Castor Oil/Poke Root Oil	Massage daily

MASTITIS

If breast feeding:

Apply mullein/lobelia salve to affected area on single breast only—nurse from other breast. Or apply calendula oil to affected breast—nurse from other breast.

PHYSIOLOGY OF MENOPAUSE

HYPOTHALMUS/PITUITARY

These glands are responsible for secretion of FSH + LH hormones (anterior pituitary gonadotrophic hormones). The purpose of FSH + LH hormone is to stimulate the ovaries to produce estrogen.

As the menopause phase begins, ovarian follicles become depleted and less estrogen is secreted. Because of a feedback loop of hormones, there is then less negative feedback on the hypothalmus and women experience and increase in GRH (Gonadotropin Releasing Hormone) and an increase in FSH (Follicle Stimulating Hormone) and a slight increase in LH (Luteal Hormone) which in tum attempts to stimulate the ovaries to secrete more estrogen.

At this time ovulation continues even though less estrogen is present. Yet women secrete the same amount of progesterone. The onset of menopause is due to a combination of ovarian aging (depletion of follicles) and extra-ovarian changes.

Depletion of follicles happens at a fairly consistent rate. At the onset of menopause, the rate of depletion accelerates—and because of the feedback loop increase of FSH hormone (which at one time caused more estrogen to be secreted from ovarian follicles) it now is involved in speeding up the depletion of follicles. So, in time, much less estrogen is secreted.

The body may produce more estrogen from sources other than ovaries before menopause and continue after menopause. Adrenals may be involved in estrogen production.

Estrogenic Herbs
Foeniculum vulgare (Fennel)
Salvia off. (Sage)
Cimicifuga racemosa (Black Cohosh)
Angelica sinensis (Dong Quai)
Anisum pimpinella (Anise)
Arctium lappa (Burdock)
Medicago sativa (Alfalfa)
Panax quiquifolia (Ginseng)

Progesterone Herbs
Glycyrrhiza glabra (Licorice)
Smilax off. (Sarsaparilla
Dioscorea villosa (Wild Yam)

MENOPAUSE

Between the ages of 45 and 55 years, ovarian tissues gradually cease to respond to stimulation by anterior pituitary gonadotrophic hormones. After menopause, a woman is unable to bear children.

During and after menopause, the secondary sex organs atrophy. The Fallopian tubes become smaller, while the uterine cycle and menstruation cease. The muscles and lining of the uterus, as well as the vaginal epithelium, reduce in thickness, while the external genitalia shrink.

Ups and downs in emotions are partly related to the fact that the ovaries cease to respond to follicle-stimulating hormone. This results in the reduction of estrogen and progesterone levels in the body. Vasomotor phenomena such as "hot flashes" (vasodilation) can produce excessive sweating and giddiness. The ovary becomes small and fibrosed, and no longer produces ripe ova. There can also be a reversal of typically female secondary sex characteristics: body fat may be redistributed, the breasts may shrink along with the internal ducts, and hair may become sparse in the axillary area (armpit) and the pubis.

ESTROGEN REPLACEMENT THERAPY

BASIC ESTROGEN REPLACEMENT *

Medicago sativa (Alfalfa Solid Extract)	1 teaspoon b.i.d.
Compounded Vitex Elixir	1 teaspoon t.i.d.
Compounded Vitex/Alfalfa	30–40 drops q.i.d.

If symptomatology is present, compound of the following herbs:

Caulophylum thalictroides (Blue Cohosh)	20 drops t.i.d.
Hyssopus officinalis (Hyssop)	20 drops t.i.d.
Scutellaria lateriflora (Skullcap)	20 drops t.i.d.
Salvia officinalis (Sage)	20 drops t.i.d.
Chamoelirium luteum (Helonias Root)	20 drops t.i.d.
Glycyrrhiza glabra (Licorice Root)	10 drops t.i.d.
Arctium lappa (Burdock Root)	20 drops t.i.d.
Dioscorea villosa (Wild Yam)	30 drops t.i.d.
Evening PrimroseOil	500 mg. t.i.d.

Take the above program for 4–6 months, then one month off before continuing for another 4–6 months.

Specific Differentiation:

Vitex agnus castus (Chaste Tree berry)	30 drops t.i.d.
Chelidonium major (Greater Celandine)	10 drops t.i.d.
Cimicifuga racemosa (Black Cohosh)	15 drops t.i.d.
Pulsatilla	5 drops t.i.d.

The above compound is to be taken when there is lability and nervous over-excitability.

Menopause Differentiation:

The following differentiations are added to the standard botanical estrogen replacement therapy cited above.

Hot Flashes
Compound:

Salvia officinalis (Sage)	20 drops
Leonurus cardiaca (Motherwort)	20 drops
Mentha piperta (Peppermint)	20 drops
Compounded Vitex/Alfalfa	40 drops q.i.d.

Osteoporosis
Avena sativa (Wild Oats)
Urtica dioica (Nettles)
Althea officinalis (Marshmallow Root)

Rumex crispus (Yellow Dock)
Equisetum officinalis (Horsetail)

> Drink 3 cups daily using liberal amounts of herbs to make strong decoction.

Manganese	2.5 mg I day
Liquid Vitamin K	5 mg/day

Blood Sugar Changes:

Compounded Devil's Club	30–40 drops q.i.d.
Arctium lappa (Burdock Root)	30 drops q.i.d.
Glycyrrhiza glabra (Licorice Root)	20 drops t.i.d.

Genito–Urinary:

Compounded Usnea/Uva Ursi (if UTI present)

> 30–60 q.i.d. or more frequently

Compound:

Helonias Root (False Unicorn)	20 drops t.i.d.
Smilax officinalis (Sarsaparilla)	20 drops t.i.d.
Aletris (True Unicorn)	20 drops t.i.d.

INFERTILITY

Compound of the following herbs:

Chamaelirium luteum (Helonias Root)	30 drops t.i.d.
Vitex agnus castus (Chaste Tree Berry)	20 drops t.i.d.
Mitchella repens (Squaw Vine)	20 drops t.i.d.
Aletris farinosa (True Unicorn)	15 drops t.i.d.
Lobelia incarnata (Lobelia)	10 drops t.i.d.
Zingiber officinalis (Ginger Root, Fresh)	10 drops t.i.d.
Octocossinol	500 mg q.i.d.
Wheat Germ Oil	1 teaspon b.i.d.

Tea prepared of the following herbs:

Urtica dioica (Nettles)

Avena sativa (Oat seed/straw)

Rubus idaeus (Raspberry leaf)

Take large amount of each herb (1 handful) and add to 2 quarts boiling water. Simmer on low for 20 minutes, turn off heat and steep overnight. In morning, strain and warm, then add 1 tablespoon He Shu Wu Tonic. Drink 1 quart daily.

PREGNANCY

THREE STAGES IN A CYCLE ENDING IN PREGNANCY

The fimbriated end of the uterine tube receives ovum at ovulation. The uterine tube also transmits spermatozoa towards the ova.

1. Fertilization
Fusion of ovum and sperm—occurs in outer third of uterine tube.

2. Cleavage
After fertilization in Fallopian tube, the fertilized ovum (zygote) undergoes several divisions. Ciliary currents and peristaltic contractions in Fallopian tube carry blastocyst into uterine secretions around the fourth to the seventh day.

3. Implantation
For a few days, the embryo gets oxygen and nutrients by diffusion from the uterine glandular secretions. The embryo sticks to lining of womb. Its surface trophoblast cells fuse with, destroy, and finally penetrate the endometrium (now called the desidua). The embryo now absorbs tissue fluids and cellular debris. Chorionic villi, finger-like projections from the embryo, invade the mother's endometrial blood vessels. The endometrium is in luteal phase, and continues to grow. No menstrual degeneration occurs. Glands are actively secreting mucus.

HERBS CONTRAINDICATED DURING PREGNANCY

BY ACTIONS:
- (US) Uterine Stimulants
- (E) Emmenogogues
- (A) Abortifacients

BY CHEMISTRY:
- (AL) Anthraquinone Laxatives
- (EO) Essential Oils
- (AK) Alkaloids
- (B) Bitter Principles

Achellia millefolium	(Yarrow)	EO, B, E
Acorus calamus	(Calamus)	B, E, US
Artemesia spp.	(Wormwood)	US, E, A, EO
Bemeris vulgaris	(Barberry)	B, AK
Capsicum spp.	(Cayenne)	EO, US
Chelidonium maius	(Celandine)	AK, B
Dryopteris filix–mas	(Male fem)	B, US

Ephedra spp.	(Ephedra)	AK, B
Foeniculum vulgare	(Fennel)	EO, US
Glycyrrhiza glabra	(Licorice)	US, E
Hydrastis canadensis	(Goldenseal)	B, AK, US
Juniperus communis	(Juniper)	EO, B
Lavendula offlcinalis	(Lavender)	EO, B
Linum usitatissimum	(Flaxseed)	US
Menthae pulegium	(Pennyroyal)	EO, US, E, A
Passiflora incarnata	(Passion Flower)	EO, US, E
Phytolacca americanium	(Poke Root)	US, E, A
Podophyllum pelatum	(Mayapple)	US, E, A, AL
Prunus serotina	(Wild Cherry)	B, US
Rhamnus spp.	(Cascara Sagrada)	E, US, AL,
Rheum spp.	(Rhubarb)	E, US, AL B
Salvia officinalis	(Sage)	EO, B, US
Sanguinaria canadensis	(Bloodroot)	AK, P, US
Tanacetum vulgare	(Tansy)	EO,B,US,E,A
Thuia occidentalis	(Thuja)	EO, US, E
Thymus vulgaris	(Thyme)	EO, US, E
Vinca rosea	(Periwinkle)	US, E
Viscum album	(Mistletoe)	US, E

HERBS TO BE USED WITH CAUTION DURING PREGNANCY

Angelica archangelica	(Angelica)
Angelica sinensis	(Dong Quai)
Arctium lappa	(Burdock)
Arctostaphylos uva ursi	(Uva Ursi)
Calendula officinalis	(Calendula)
Hydrocotyle asiatica	(Gotu Kola)
Hypericum perforatum	(St. John's Wort)
Hyssopus officinalis	(Hyssop)
Leonurus cardiaca	(Motherwort)
Marrubium vulgare	(Horehound)
Matricaria chamonublia	(German Chamomile)
Medicago sativa	(Alfalfa)
Melissa officinalis	(Lemon Balm)
Mentha piperita	(Peppermint)
Plantago spp.	(Plantain)
Silybum marianum	(Milk Thistle)
Tanacetum parthenium	(Feverfew)
Trigoneua fuenumgraecum	(Fennugreek)
Urtica dioica	(Nettles)
Zingiber officinalis	(Ginger)

USEFUL HERBS DURING PREGNANCY

Caulophyllum thalictroides	(Blue Cohosh)★
Chamaelirum luteum	(False Unicorn)
Crataegus spp.	(Hawthorn)
Dioscorea villosa	(Wild Yam)
Mitchella repens	(Squaw Vine)
Rubus idaeus	(Red Raspberry)
Scutellaria lateriflora	(Skullcap)
Taraxacum officinalis	(Dandelion)
Urtica dioica	(Nettles)
Viburnum opulus	(Cramp Bark)
Viburnum prunifolium	(Black Haw)

★During Last Trimester Only

BOTANICAL THERAPIES FOR CONDITIONS DURING PREGNANCY

Threatened Miscarriage
Compound:
> *Viburnum prunifolium* (Black Haw)
> *Chamaelirium luteum* (False Unicorn)
> *Cimifuga racemosa* (Black Cohosh)
> *VIburnum opulus* (Cramp Bark)
> > Use 20–30 drops each q.i.d.

Anemia
Decoction (tea) of the following herbs:
> *Rubus idaeus* (Red Raspberry leaf)
> *Taraxacum officinalis* (Dandelion Root)
> *Urtica dioica* (Nettles)
> *Avena sativa* (Oats)
> *Rumex crispus* (Yellow Dock)
> > Drink 16–24 oz./day of the above tea

Yellow Dock Extract	30 drops t.i.d.
Compounded Nutritional Elixir	1 teaspoon b.i.d./t.i.d.
Chlorella algae	1 teaspoon in water b.i.d.
Folic Acid	

Nausea

Gentiana Lutea (Gentian)	20 drops t.i.d.
Filependula ulmarea (Meadowsweet)	20 drops t.i.d.
Foeniculim vulgare (Fennel)	20 drops t.i.d.
Cinnamonum aromaticum (Cinnamon)	20 drops t.i.d.
Zinginber officinalis (Ginger)	5 drops t.i.d.
Liquid Vitamin K	5 mg/day

Constipation
• Stewed Figs. Simmer 10 calimyrna figs in 16 oz. water for 10 minutes. Steep overnight. In the morning, drink

warm fig juice and eat figs throughout the day.
- Oat Milk. Soak freshly ground oats in water overnight, 3 pounds water to 1 pound oats. In the morning, strain through cheesecloth, saving milk of oats. Warm oat milk and add fig juice or prune juice to sweeten. Also add 30 drops *Glycyrrhiza glabra* (Licorice Extract) to oat milk.
- Pure Extra Virgin Olive Oil–Take 1 Tablespoon 3x daily, between meals.
- Do yoga stretching exercises/abdominal stretches daily.

Compound:

Rumex crispus (Yellow Dock)	15 drops t.i.d.
Taraxacum officinalis (Dandelion Root)	15 drops t.i.d.
Dioscorea villosa (Wild Yam)	10 drops t.i.d.
Ulmus Rubra (Slippery Elm)	1/2–1 teaspoon t.i.d.
Pimpinella anisum (Anise)	10 drops t.i.d.

Add the above mixture to Compounded Psyllium Husk Powder. Take 1 teaspoon in large glass of warm water. Add herbal extracts above and take 1x/day.

Hemorrhoids
- Rub or inject with a small syringe into rectum comfrey-compounded oil b.i.d.
- Take warm sitz baths each evening before bed for 15–20 minutes.

Urinary Tract Infections (UTI)
Compounded Usnea/Uva Ursi

40–60 drops every 2 hours
or until infection subsides.
(Note: Do not drink cranberry juice at this time.)

Hypertension
Compound:

Crataegus (Hawthorn Supreme)	40–60 drops q.i.d.
Taraxacum (Dandelion Root/Leaf)	20–30 drops q.i.d.
Tilia spp. (Linden)	20 drops q.i.d.
Matricaria chamonulia (Chamomile)	20 drops q.i.d.

Drink warm water every 15 minutes throughout the day.

Leg Cramps
Compounded Calcium Elixir

1 teaspoon b.i.d. when cramps appear

Viburnum opulus (Cramp Bark)	20 drops
Viburnum prunifolium (Black Haw)	20 drops

Take the above herbs t.i.d. when cramps appear.

NATUROPATHIC
Desk Reference

DISORDERS OF IMMEDIATE-TYPE HYPER-SENSITIVITY

Asthmatic Reactions
Allergies
Hives
Urticaria
Reactive Dermatitis
Reactive Inflammatory Arthritis
Reactive Psoriasis
Irritable Bowel Syndrome

BOTANICAL MATERIA MEDICA

Achillea millefolium
 (Yarrow)
Angelica sinensis (Dong
 Quai)
Catechu nigrum (Black
 Catechu)
Camellia thea (Green Tea)
Curcuma longa (Turmeric)
Echinacea spp. (Echinacea)
Ephedra sinensis (Ma
 Huang)
Euphrasia off. (Eyebright)
Ginkgo biloba (Ginkgo)
Glycyrrhiza glabra (Licorice)

Grindelia robusta
 (Grindelia)
Harpagophytum
 procumbens (Devil's
 Claw)
Hydrastis canadensis
 (Goldenseal)
Lobelia inflata (Lobelia)
Myrica cerifera (Bayberry)
Silybum marianum (Milk
 Thistle)
Urtica dioica (Stinging
 Nettles)

THE ALLERGIC RESPONSE SYNDROME

The allergy syndrome, now being referred to medically as
disorders of immediate type hypersensitivity includes a broad
spectrum of health imbalances which include asthma,
allergies (pollen, animal dander, molds, airborne pollutants,
etc.), hives, urticaria, reactive dermatitis, food allergies,
psoriasis, reactive inflammatory arthritis, irritable bowel
syndrome, spastic colon, colitis anaphylaxis shock syndrome,
etc. Primary sites of reactivity include the skin, mucous
membranes, and joints. The reactivities occur as a result of a
hypersensitivity and instability of the secretory immune
system which partly consists of the mucous membrane
throughout the body.

Imbedded in these tissues are immune cells called *mast cells*
which become unstable and eventually degranulate when
they are repeatedly contacted by allergens originating either
from the environment or as a biproduct of metabolism.

HYPE 1

Eventually inflammatory histamines and other inflammatory substances "leak" through the membranes, evoking the inflammatory response. Mucous membranes may become irritated and swollen and secrete excess mucous. Skin may become irritated, itchy, and develop hives or urticaria or break out in psoriatic lesions. Joints may become painful and inflamed. Bowels may become irritated and spastic, with resulting malabsorption. All of the above reactivities occur as a result of pathways of inflammation becoming activated through the release of inflammatory substances from mast cells.

FOOD ALLERGIES

Cytotoxic Reactions

Tissue injury occurs when IgG or IgM antibodies bind to cell-bound antigens. Antigen-antibody binding can eventually cause cell destruction where the antigen is bound.

Immune Complex–Mediated Reactions

Resulting tissue injury is due to binding of antigens to antibodies, which eventually deposit in tissues. These reactions result from circulating antigenic complexes and vasoactive amines found in food.

The resolution of this immediate type of hypersensitivity and food allergies includes the following approaches:

- Stabilize mast cells
- Improve mucous membrane integrity
- Improve integrity of gut and intestinal mucosa
- Enhance the adrenal response towards the activation of inflammatory pathways
- Protect liver integrity and improve the ability of the liver to clear these allergens from the system
- Provide immune support

The botanical approach to this resolution includes largely the use of *flavonoids* derived from many specific plants. Four important flavonoids (quercetin, curcumin, catechin, silymarin) are derived from the use of the following plants: Turmeric root, Catechu, and Milk Thistle seed. These plants significantly improve mast cell and mucous membrane integrity and protect hepatocytes, while improving the ability of the liver to clear antigens from the system. The following botanical protocol has been developed as a thorough treatment for all disorders of immediate type hypersensitivity.

BOTANICAL THERAPY FOR IMMEDIATE-TYPE HYPERSENSITIVITY DISORDER

Compounded Turmeric/Catechu
    30-40 drops 3-4x daily between meals for 4-6 months

Fresh Nettles Extract
    30-50 drops 3-4x daily 1 month prior to onset of allergy season and continue for 4-6 months

Compounded Echinacea   30-40 drops q.i.d.

Licorice Root Solid Extract
    1/8-1/4 teaspoon 2x daily for 2-4 weeks

Compounded Bitters Elixir
    1/2-1 teaspoon 3x daily in a small amount of warm water before meals for 4-6 months

Compounded Psyllium Husk Powder
    1 heaping teaspoon in a full glass of warm water, 2x daily for 3-4 months

Compounded Vitamin C Elixir   1 t b.i.d.

Linseed Oil   1T b.i.d.

Differentiations:

Compounded Eyebright/Bayberry   20-30 drops 3x daily for 2 weeks
    NOTE: To be used only if allergic response includes excessive mucous secretions and exudations

Ma Huang   30-40 drops 3-4x daily for 2 weeks
    NOTE: To be used only if bronchial constriction is present

Compound for Asthma:

Grindelia robusta (Grindelia)   30 drops q.i.d.
Glycyrrhiza glabra (Licorice)   20 drops q.i.d.
Lobelia inflata (Lobelia)   10 drops q.i.d.
Compounded Vitamin C Elixir   1/2 t q.i.d.
    Add the above to warm water or Green tea
Green tea   Drink 2-4 cups daily

Compounded Turmeric/Catechu

Contents:

Curcuma longa (Turmeric)
Catechu nigra (Black Catechu)
Grindelia robusta (Grindelia)
Glycyrrhiza glabra (Licorice)
Rosa rugosa (Rose Hips)
Scutellaria baicalensis (Chinese Skullcap)
Ginkgo biloba (Ginkgo)
Harpagophytum procumberis (Devils Claw)
Achellia millefolium (Yarrow)
Lobelia inflata (Lobelia)

Compounded Eyebright/Bayberry

Contents:

Euphrasia off. (Eyebright)
Myrica cerifera (Bayberry)
Hydrastis canadensis (Goldenseal)
Acorus calamus (Calamus)
Urtica dioica (Nettles)

Compounded Bitters Elixir

Contents:

Curcuma longa (Turmeric)
Emblica off (Indian Gooseberry)
Silybum marianum (Milk Thistle)
Dioscorea villosa (Wild Yam)
Gentiana lutea (Gentian)
Aeorus calamus (Calamus)
Foeniculum vulgare (Fennel)
Elettaria cardaimonum (Cardamon)

Compounded Psyllium Husk Powder

Contents:

Plantago ovata (Psyllium)
Triphala concentrate
Althaea off. (Marshmallow)
Glycyrrhiza glabra (Licorice)
Zingiber off. (Ginger)

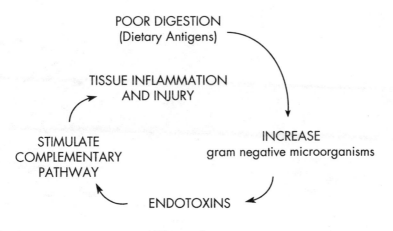

Diagram 1

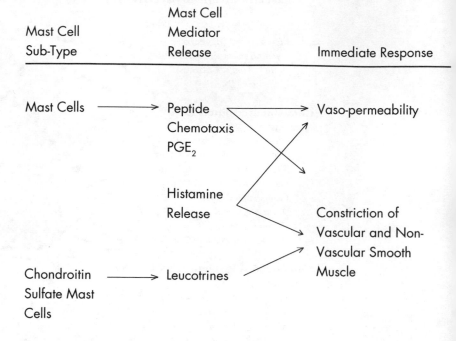

Diagram 2

**Stress, Adaptogens, and the Immune System:
Harmonizing the Chemistry of Man
with the Chemistry of Nature**

•••••••••••••••••••••••••••••

NATUROPATHIC
Desk Reference

•••••••••••••••••••••••••••

A study of the teaching and writing of some of the most
respected physicians, teachers, and practitioners of natural
methods of healing reveals the following five **principals of
nature cure**:

NERVE INTEGRITY
BLOOD & LYMPHATIC INTEGRITY
CIRCULATION
ASSIMILATION
ELIMINATION

These five fundamental principals of health, if operating in a
balanced way within the physiology, will result in the
improvement of the **vital force** of the individual.

NERVE INTEGRITY

To have healthy nerve integrity is to have a strong and
balanced nerve system, nerve cells, nerve sheath, brain cells,
and spinal cord. All information and electrical impulses are
coordinated and carried out through the nerve system
network. The nerve system is supported and maintained
nutritionally by several fundamental elementals, which
include calcium, magnesium, sodium, potassium, phosphorus, silicon, iron, and iodine. The elemental forms of
these minerals as they occur naturally in the vegetative and
animal kingdom carry the wisdom of nature's intelligence so
that they target and align to the designated complementary
receptors in the body.

Calcium: "The Great Builder"
Calcium and its elemental forms such as calcium phosphate,
calcium chloride, and calcium fluoride are essential for healthy
nerve, brain, and structural integrity. With elemental calcium
new tissues and cells remain strong and vital. Calcium maintains the connective network within the body and supports
the solidarity of the body. Elemental forms of calcium in foods
and herbs are best found in seeds such as sesame, sunflower,
and pumpkin, as well as almonds, figs, dark greens, oats, rice,
barley, carrots, and seaweeds. Excellent herbal sources of
elemental calcium are oats, horsetail, skullcap, hawthorn berry,
gotu kola, and stinging nettles.

Magnesium: "The Great Relaxer"

Magnesium in it's elemental form as it naturally occurs in plants is considered to be the finest relaxer, tranquilizer, and laxative in nature.

Magnesium brings relaxation to an agitated nerve system and soothes irritation to the tissues and cells associated with nerve function. It also relieves constipation and irritation to the bowels, resulting from an over–stressed physiology. Elemental forms of magnesium in foods and herbs are best found in many orange and yellow foods such as carrots, yellow squash, sweet potato, and yellow corn, as well as black mission figs, and raw goat's milk. Herbal sources of magnesium include Gotu Kola, skullcap, horsetail, alfalfa, nettles, hawthorn berry, and wild oat seed.

Sodium: "The Youth Element"

Sodium in its naturally occurring form is considered to bring youthfulness to the body's tissues, membrane linings, and joints. Sodium is essential for healthy digestion and supple capillaries and arteries. It is necessary to maintain flexibility and mobility in the joints. Without proper sodium the joints would stiffen and calcify prematurely. Without proper sodium the lining of the stomach would not secrete the necessary enzymes for healthy digestion.

The Sun is considered the sodium star, so all fruits and vegetables which are ripened by the sun contain ample amounts of sodium. Other significant sources of sodium include seaweed such as kelp, dulse, and nori, as well as black mission figs, whey, celery, and raw goat milk. Herbal sources of sodium include alfalfa, chlorella, spirulina, stinging nettles, and raspberry leaf.

Potassium: "The Great Alkalizer"

Potassium salts as they occur naturally in foods bring alkalinity to the blood chemistry. Potassium neutralizes acids in blood chemistry which build from incorrect metabolism of unsuitable foods for the constitution. Potassium, when in balance, prevents the growth of cysts, fibroids, and other benign growths. Without potassium balance, the nervous system may become agitated, thoughts become disturbed and the entire psycho-physiological balance is upset. All fresh fruits and vegetables contain ample amounts of potassium, especially figs, celery, dandelion greens, and other dark green leafy vegetables. Herbal sources of potassium include stinging nettles, dandelion, alfalfa, seaweed, parsley, and chickweed.

Phosphorus: "The Light Bearer"

Phosphorus feeds both the brain and nerve cells as well as the bones. Brain and nerve phosphorus is obtained largely through animal derivatives and single cell algae, while bone phosphorus can be obtained through seeds and nuts. Without adequate phosphorus to feed the constitution, one may feel dull and lethargic and may lack radiance. One's bones may be deficient and early structural disorders may arise. A vegetarian must maintain spiritual and emotional balance in order to hold adequate phosphorus in the system. Sources of phosphorus derived from fish and poultry, seeds, nuts, and whole grains can adequately keep balance in the physiology.

Silicon: "The Magnetic Element"

Silicon in it's naturally occurring form feeds the nerve cells, nerve sheath, hair, nails, skin, eyes, teeth, brain cells, and tissues. Silica brings magnetism to the nerves, brings radiance to the skin, luster to the hair, builds strong teeth and nails, and brings balance to the emotional system. A person lacking silica will be tense, irritable, rough, appear cold and difficult to get to know, lack luster, and generally feels on edge much of the time. While a person who is rich in silica will sparkle, radiate joy and harmony, express dynamism in personality, attract others, show luster in hair, eyes, teeth, and nails, and generally be very magnetic. People are naturally drawn to silica-rich people. Without adequate silica, one remains lonely and feels depleted. Silica is naturally found in the outer husks of whole grains, seeds, and nuts. Rich herbal sources of silica include horsetail, wild oats, dandelion leaf, onions, alfalfa, and stinging nettles.

Iron: "The Frisky Horse Element"

Iron is the element which builds vigor and stamina into the constitution. Iron gives strength and virility. Without adequate iron the blood becomes depleted and one feels weak, anemic, and frail. Iron from inorganic sources may not be absorbed well into the tissues and can cause constipation, yeast overgrowth, and can lead to auto—intoxication. Iron attracts oxygen into the constitution and gives mental energy and clarity of mind. Naturally occurring sources of iron are figs, raisins, dark green leafy vegetables, black cherries, chlorella, spirulina, stinging nettles, dandelion leaf, raspberry leaf, alfalfa, chickweed, parsley, and red clover. Herbal iron tonics, inclusive of the herbs, are best assimilated when gentian root is added to the formula—due to it's nascent oxygen which aids in the assimilation of iron.

Iodine: "The Emotional Metabolizer Element"

Iodine is the element which feeds the thyroid gland and maintains metabolic and emotional balance throughout the body. Without adequate iodine, the thyroid gland may become dysfunctional and lead to metabolic changes. Every emotion which we experience is processed through the thyroid gland. Without adequate iodine, emotional instability may arise and the nervous system may feel distraught.

Ample sources of iodine are found in seaweeds such as kelp, dulse, and nori, as well as onions and black walnut hulls and nuts.

Each of the preceding chemical elements is intimately connected to healthy nerve integrity in it's own way. When the body is in chemical balance, the nerve cells and tissues maintain sufficient vitality to eliminate metabolic wastes and to coordinate all electrical and nerve impulses throughout the system.

BLOOD AND LYMPHATIC INTEGRITY

The two main bodily fluids, the blood and lymph, require proper chemical and metabolic balance. When the blood and lymph fluids are laden with toxic wastes, other organ and tissue functions become impeded. One simple nature cure method of maintaining healthy blood and lymph fluids is to drink regular warm water throughout the day. Warm water keeps the body's channels open, permitting vital energy to flow through the system. Warm water also enables wastes to soften and loosen from impacted areas so that they may be eliminated freely. Warm water also enables toxins to be flushed out of the system throughout the day so that one's energy may be sustained evenly.

Another nature cure method to enhance blood and lymphatic integrity is to do regular morning dry skin brushing upon rising. Dry skin brushing invigorates the peripheral circulation and mobilizes toxic lymph to drain into eliminative channels for better elimination. Alterative herbal therapies, which alter processes of waste and nutrition through metabolism, are effective in enhancing blood and lymphatic integrity. Some effective alterative therapies include Scudders Alterative Compound, Compounded Red Clover, Compounded Hoxsey/Red Clover, and Compounded Echinacea /Red Root (See the herbal dispensatory section for specific information on these alterative therapies).

CIRCULATION

All nutrients are carried through the system within the circulatory system. To feed the cells and tissues properly, the organs of circulation—the heart, lungs, and spleen— must be functioning healthfully. Fresh clean air, exercise, and deep breathing exercises promote healthy circulation. Constitutional herbal therapies which promote healthy circulation include Compounded Hawthorn, ginkgo leaf, ginger root, prickly ash bark, cayenne pepper, siberian ginseng, as well as the herbs cited above.

ASSIMILATION

Real assimilation begins when the sun's influence comes in contact with the body at dawn. The sun is the fire element in nature and as it grows stronger in the sky, it builds the fires of appetite and digestion. When the sun is highest in the sky, digestion and assimilation are at their strongest. Therefore, it makes sense naturopathically to eat one's largest meal during the noon hour.

Some people believe that "you are what you eat." This is perhaps only a partial truth. What may be more truthful is "you are what you assimilate." All eastern medicine (Ayurvedic and Chinese) is founded on the premise that health is born of strong digestion.

Another value of assimilation is born of our experiences. Every experience that we entertain—every thought, every like and dislike, every instinct, every emotion, literally every impulse of the breath of life—gets assimilated into our psycho-physiology and creates our physical body. Our body is the end product of our experiences. Daily experiences get metabolized and transmuted into physical matter. Therefore it is essential to cultivate healthy assimilation of our daily life by creating routines which are in balance with the operating principles and forces of nature.

ELIMINATION

We find that if the previous four principles of nature cure are attended to properly and routinely, the byproduct will be healthy elimination through all the eliminative channels. There are six major channels of elimination—the skin, kidneys, bowel, liver, lungs, and lymph. With a healthy routine, fresh air, clean water, healthy foods, graceful eating of food, exercise, and life-supporting environments, all channels of elimination should be impacted favorably. It should not be necessary to resort to laxatives of any kind to move one's bowels. Constipation results from improper digestion and improper maintenance of nerve force.

When all five principles of nature cure are operating freely and routinely, the most fundamental result will be the revitalization of the vital force within the body.

FORMULA FOR VITALITY: RESTORATION OF THE VITAL FORCE

Power and vitality result from the elimination of obstructing wastes in the body and secondly from assimilating "nature" into the physiology. Vital force is the key ingredient for health and longevity. All physio–medical therapy attempts to restore the vital force. When vital force is strong, immunity is strong. In Ayurvedic medicine it is said that when digestion is at its peak, then "ojas" is produced as the most refined substance of digestion. Ojas is the nectar of life—it sustains life. When ojas is strong then one gets "bala." Bala is an Ayurvedic term which is translated to mean strength and immunity. From this perspective it is clear that digestion is of key importance for vital force, which is of key importance for immunity from disease.

THE ADAPTIVE SYNDROME

Adaptogenic Medicine:
Strengthening the Powers of Resistance

The term "adaptogenic medicine" was first coined by a Russian scientist, Lazarev, who referred to medically effective substances which he called adaptogens as substances which put the body into a state of non–specific heightened resistance in order to better resist stress and adapt to extraordinary challenges. Dr. Hans Selye, a Swedish scientist who won a Nobel Prize for his work on stress, formulated what he called the General Adaptive Syndrome. It was Selye who said that there is no stressful situation in life, only a stressful response. How we respond to stress determines the effect that stress will have on us.

Selye felt the limiting factor which determined our adaptive capacity and resulting immunity was what he coined the "Adaptations Energy" of the body. He felt that one's powers of resistance and resistance reserves are not inexhaustible, and that they diminish when the body is continuously exposed to extreme stress—the consequences being misadaptation, lowered immunity, and the onset of disease.

Selye's General Adaptive Syndrome provided for three distinct phases:

1. **The "Alarm Reaction"**
   This is the first phase, which is a response to the exposure to stressful stimuli. This phase sets in usually within a few minutes to several hours after exposure to the stress. Sympathetic nerve changes occur which represent the body's response to stress; generally, the body begins a degenerative process which invariably raises the non–specific resistance capacity.

2. **The "Stage of Resistance"**
    If the stressor prevails upon the body, the second phase sets in. The body may respond with a heightened capacity of resistance to the stressor. In this phase the Adaptive Energy is sufficient enough to bring about a normalization of the changes which originated during the first phase. Here the body becomes increasingly resistant until optimal adaptation is achieved.

3. **The "Stage of Exhaustion"**
    If the stressor is permitted to expose the body and goes beyond a certain limit, the "Adaptive Energy" becomes depleted. Here the resistance of the body is exhausted. The capacity for adaptation is lost. In this phase the organs and cells and tissues begin to break down and eventually disease begins to set in.

Naturally, one would want to recognize the impact of a stressor and change the environment so that the powers of resistance remain strong. A Russian scientist, Brekhman, coined the term "Adaptogenic Medicine" recognizing that there were substances in nature which could sustain the powers of resistance when stressors continue to expose the body. Brekhman saw that in the plant kingdom the were specific plants which had the capacity to exert an "Adaptogenic Effect" upon the physiology. He referred to these plants as adaptogens. He summarized the concept of plant adaptogens in the following way:

1. The plant must show a non–specific effect (raising the powers of resistance to stressors of a physical, chemical, or emotional nature).

2. The plant must normalize the physiology—it must restore balance and equilibrium even in the presence of pathological conditions.

3. The plant must be non–toxic and harmless to any organ or tissue within the body.

Thus adaptogens are plant substances capable of strengthening the non–specific powers of resistance to stress, capable of raising the general performance capacity during stressful exposure, and capable of preventing disease which may develop due to over–stressing the body.

HERBS KNOWN FOR THEIR ADAPTOGENIC EFFECTS

Siberian Ginseng *(Eleutherococcus senticosus)*

This plant contains compounds known as eleutherosides which are primarily responsible for the adaptogenic attributes which it exhibits. There also exists immunomodulating polysaccharides (long-chain sugar molecules) found in the root. Studies show that when taken regularly the adaptogenic effects of Siberian Ginseng permit a greater resistance to adverse conditions such as excessive work load and exercise, exposure to pollutants, exposure to excessive noise and environmental stress, and stress due to pathogenesis, including cancer, arthritis, diabetes, hypertension, heart disease, respiratory disorders, nerve disorders, as well as a variety of other ailments. Although Siberian Ginseng may not be a cure for any of these pathogenic conditions, it has been shown to bring more balance and equilibrium to the physiology when affected by these ailments. Generally, Siberian Ginseng is found useful for anyone undergoing a stress overload and seems to be more effective if taken cumulatively over a period of 4–6 months. Generally if taken over this time Siberian Ginseng will exhibit marked anti–stress effects, endocrine effects (lowers cholesterol, increases corticosteroids, increases secretions of male reproductive glands), and anabolic effects (improves protein synthesis in liver, pancreas, and adrenal cortex).

American Ginseng *(Panax quinquifolius)*

This plant contains a group of saponin compounds known as ginsenosides. Ginsenosides in the roots of American Ginseng have been shown to have an adaptogenic effect similar to that of Siberian Ginseng. The General Adaptive Energies of the body are strengthened, bringing a greater resistance to stressful stimuli. American Ginseng has also been shown to exhibit anti-tumor, anti–viral, anti–oxidant, metabolic, and endocrine properties. It has been shown to reduce fatigue, strengthen adrenal response, enhance reproductive performance, improve liver metabolism and enhance immunity. The Chinese regard American Ginseng as a Yin Tonic, reducing heat in the digestive and respiratory systems. For this reason it is considered more favorable for individuals with a hotter constitution.

Schizandra Berry *(Schizandra chinensis)*

Schizandra Berries originate in China and are considered to possess general adaptogen activity, regulating a variety of body functions and improving the body's response to stress. Schizandra exhibits three ranges of actions. Firstly, it shows marked anti–hepatotoxic and hepatoprotective action. In this respect it protects liver cells, promotes regeneration of hepatocytes, enhances liver detoxification, and is effective in the treatment of chronic hepatitis and cirrhosis. Secondly, it shows marked metabolic action, increasing hepatic glycogen content and relieving fatty degeneration of the liver. Thirdly, its adaptogenic action is strong in improving overall response to stress, improving sensory response, and strengthening central and peripheral nerve systems.

Ashwaganda Root *(Withania somnifera)*
In Ayurvedic medicine the root is said to "protect the organism from illness through maintaining the healthy balance of physical energies." It is considered to be a tonic in a similar sense as that of Ginseng. Like other adaptogens, Ashwaganda exhibits an anti–stress effect, an immunomodulatory effect, it enhances both short and long term memory, and exhibits anti–inflammatory properties.

Astragalus Root *(Astragalus membranaceus)*
In Chinese medicine, Astragalus is considered to be a Chi Tonic. It has the capacity to build the energy reserves in the body while at the same time exhibiting several anti–stress properties. Astragalus Root enhances liver metabolism of endogenous and exogenous toxins. It shows a cardiotonic effect with the capacity of lowering blood pressure. It possesses marked anti–microbial properties especially against Shigella spp., Streococcus haemolyticus, and Staphylococcus aureus. It influences the kidney meridian and has been shown to improve urine flow and to be effective in urinary and bladder infections. If taken cumulatively, especially with Chinese *Ligustrum lucidum* berries, it shows marked anti–tumor properties.

Other plants which have been well studied for their adaptogenic effects include Holy Basil *(Ocimum sanctum)*, Reishi mushroom *(Ganoderma lucidum)*, and Gotu Kola *(Centella asiatica)*. Other plants with less specific adaptogenic properties yet marked immunostimulating properties and immunomodulating properties include species of Echinacea *(Echinacea angustifolia, Echinacea purpurea,* and *Echinacea pallida)*.

IMMUNE-ENHANCING PROPERTIES OF ECHINACEA

Echinacea is considered a non–specific (adaptogenic) stimulant to the immune system, effecting a variety of viral and bacterial conditions influencing the secretory immune system. In this respect, Echinacea is recognized as a secretory immune stimulant influencing the mucous membranes, skin, and lymphatic system. The secretory immune system is recognized as the initial line of defense. Echinacea spp. contain a complex of different compounds responsible for their immune-enhancing effects. According to Christopher Hobbes in his monograph on Echinacea, much of the claims for Echinacea include stimulation of leukocytes, inhibition of the enzyme hyaluronidase, mild anti–biotic activity, anti–inflammatory activity, stimulation of the adrenal cortex, stimulation of the properdin/ complement system, interferon–like activity, stimulation of phagocytosis (general cellular immunity), anti–viral activity, and increased production of fibroblasts.

During conceptual stages of viral infection, Echinacea can be very effective in frequent and large doses for preventing infection by inhibiting the enzyme hyaluronidase from breaking down the cell membrane and also by strengthening the cell membrane directly. Other secretory infections such as urinary tract infections, respiratory infections, sinus infections, ear infections, and tonsillitis—all respond swiftly and convincingly to frequent and large doses of Echinacea at the onset of the infectious stage.

Adaptogenic and Immune–Enhancing Compounds
(See herbal dispensatory section for specific uses)

Compounded Ginseng/Schizandra
Compounded Siberian Ginseng Tonic
Compounded Wild Ginseng
Compounded Gotu Kola
Compounded Rejuvenative Elixir
Compounded Smilax/Damiana
Compounded Vitamin C Elixir
Compounded Echinacea

Index

Index

Index

Index

Index

INFORMATION REQUEST FORM

Please send me subscription information about the forthcoming *Protocol Journal of Botanical Medicines,* upon which the preceding botanical protocols are based.

Name

Affiliation

Address

City   State   ZIP

Daytime Phone #

Please check the following categories relevant to your work:

❑ Naturopathic Doctor   ❑ Medical Herbalist

❑ Alternative Health Practitioner   ❑ Medical Doctor

❑ Herbal/Botanical Educator   ❑ Nurse/Midwife

❑ Interested Layperson   ❑ Other _____

Please tear out this form and return to:

Kivakí Press
Protocol Journal Dept.
585 East 31st Street
Durango, CO 81301

❑ I would like to receive information on other Kivakí titles.